9

OAK LAWN PUBLIC LIBRARY

3 1186 00509 9205

A Guide to a Naturally Healthy Bird
Nutrition, Feeding, and Natural Healing Methods for Parrots

by Alicia McWatters, M.S.

W9-CNA-184

Cover photo: Congo African Grey
"Tiffany"

Published by Safe Goods

/

OCT 12 1998
OAK LAWN LIBRARY

A Guide to a Naturally Healthy Bird
Nutrition, Feeding, and Natural Healing Methods for Parrots
by Alicia McWatters, M.S.

Cover photo: Congo African Grey

Copyright© 1997 by Alicia McWatters
All Rights Reserved

No part of this book may be reproduced in any form without the written consent
of the publisher

ISBN 1-884820-21-2-15895
Library of Congress Catalog Card Number 97-69046
Printed in the United States of America

A Guide to a Naturally Healthy Bird is not intended as medical advice. It is
written solely for informational and educational purposes. Please consult a health
professional should the need for one be indicated.

Published by Safe Goods
283 East Canaan Rd.
East Canaan, CT 06024
(860)-824-5301

Foreword

Holistic medicine and a natural lifestyle has seen a remarkable groundswell of popularity in the past few years. The American Medical Association estimates that one of four health appointments made yearly are for practitioners of alternative medicine. Herbal medicine is the single most popular form of medicine world-wide according to the World Health Organization.

What is causing this trend? The belief that modern Western medicine can cure everything has been shattered. For many of us, we have watched with helplessness and frustration while friends and family members have suffered from a multitude of chronic diseases. We have also seen that Western medicine has done little for them. We have been frustrated while we watched the same things happen to our companion animals. We may know people who have recovered from some debilitating illness after being treated by an Oriental Medical Doctor, Chiropractor, Homeopath or Naturopath.

After all of these wonderful benefits we receive ourselves from this natural life style, we want the same for our companion animals. A number of excellent books have been written for dogs, cats and farm animals. However, until now, there has been no book covering birds. This is the first text, as far as I know, that is written entirely about natural health and medicine for our feathered friends, and is a welcome addition to my library!

Alicia McWatters has done a wonderful job in writing this book and should be commended for this work. She has used the methods she describes in this book on her own rather extensive flock of birds and has seen these therapies and diets in action resulting in a much healthier flock. She writes with knowledge, love and compassion about this subject which obviously is her life's calling. Health, healing and medicine is not just about antibiotics, surgery and vaccines. It is about preventive medicine, nurturing the body's vital forces, respecting nature and finding ways to help the body heal itself. Alicia knows this and conveys the meaning of this throughout the book. Many of the concepts contained herein are difficult, yet she covers them in such understandable terms that even those new to medicine, birds and natural health will enjoy reading these pages.

-Dave McCluggage, D.V.M., B.S., I.V.A.S. Certified Veterinary Acupuncturist, Chaparral Animal Health Center, Longmont, CO

Acknowledgments

First of all, I would like to express my gratitude to all the scientists, physicians, and researchers who have devoted vast amounts of time in discovering the benefits of nutrients in foods, nutritional supplements, and natural medicine. I am grateful for the aviculturists, veterinarians, herbalists, and many other educators who have shared their valuable knowledge and made it widely available to others.

I am very fortunate to have a family who encouraged my interest in the field of nutrition and have been a constant source of inspiration and love. I am particularly grateful to my husband Bruce, for without his support and patience throughout all the hours I spent putting this material together, this book would not have been possible. I am also blessed to have two wonderful sons, Travis (8) and Tyler (5) who were extremely patient and understanding of the commitment and time it took for mommy to write this book. My family's continued support has made the writing of this book a reality.

I am very lucky to share my life with so many wonderful parrot friends. My days are richer by their beauty, their companionship, and their love.

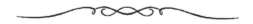

Introduction

This book is devoted to teaching you how to obtain superior health for your birds through natural feeding and natural medicines. My interest in natural health began several years ago when I became disenchanted with many of the drug treatments being used in veterinary medicine. Their repeated failure to cure illness and disease, led me to the study of nutrition and alternative treatments as tools to prevent and cure the health problems our pets experienced. I believe synthetic drugs are dangerous and often more so than the disease itself. While not every disease can be treated in a natural way and certain conditions will require conventional medicines, many of the illnesses we find our birds predisposed to, are nutritionally based and therefore diet and nutrition play an enormous role in their recovery from illness. I have found a holistic approach to health to be very effective for ameliorating many common ailments, preventing disease, and achieving optimum wellness.

I hope the advice and information on the pages that follow, will assist you in becoming more independent and knowledgeable when caring for your birds; however, I do not recommend you diagnose illness at home. If symptoms are suggestive of an illness then consulting with a holistic veterinarian experienced with nutrition and alternative medicine is advised. Resources and references are provided so that you may find additional information.

Remember that disease occurs for predictable reasons and often because the diet is deficient and nutritional solutions are overlooked. There are no mystery diseases. I believe that most diseases are the result of malnutrition and environmental adversities. You can protect your birds from disease before it starts, through proper nutrition and a healthy, stress-free environment. May your birds' health be enhanced and their lives be extended as a result of a natural diet and a healthy lifestyle.

Table of Contents

Chapter 1
Nutrition For Birds

"Let thy food be thy medicine and thy medicine be thy food"
--Hippocrates (460-377 BC)

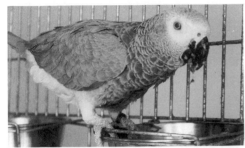

The question is often asked, "What is the proper food for birds?" Well, in the wild, our parrots, who are primarily herbivorous, find their own foods to nourish and sustain life and these foods are the living material produced by our planet Earth. Our birds are biologically adapted to fresh raw foods which, depending upon the bird species, are mainly consumed in the form of simple and complex carbohydrates (nuts, seeds, flower nectar, pollen, blossoms, berries, fruits, leaf buds, roots, vegetable matter, along with other live foods, such as, insects, larvae, and small vertebrae). In nature, food predates the eater; not the other way around. In the wild, there are no microwaves, ovens, extruders, or grain mills, etc. All life was sustained eating natural foods from natural sources. Nothing more, nothing less.

Following this logic, I feed my birds a diet as close to nature as possible and I have created a special home-prepared diet for them, made-up of all natural ingredients. This diet consists of a large variety of organically grown fruits, vegetables, legumes, grains, and seeds. In addition, I include a few natural supplements. While we cannot mimic what our birds would eat in the wild, this type of diet closely resembles the composition of the natural foods that would be found in their native habitat. The substances in fresh foods exist in an astounding complex balance that can't be reproduced in a highly processed synthetic food product. Therefore, it is my belief that serving fresh or minimally processed foods is the best way to assure that our birds are receiving the many nutrients that they require for optimum health.

Natural real foods are the ones which are inextricably linked to the life they support. There is an abundance of vitamins, minerals, enzymes, amino acids, essential fatty acids, and many other chemicals in a natural food, such as an apple, a tomato, or a floret of broccoli.

Cooking, refining, or heating to high temperatures changes the chemical and nutrient form of the food and it no longer contains the same value as it did in its original form. Vitamins and minerals are fractionated and many nutrients are completely denatured. Cooking foods kills the enzymes necessary for digestion and to perform important tasks which keep your bird's body healthy and disease-free. The risks involved with the long-term feeding of a poor diet will sooner or later result in decreased resistance to disease, digestive and degenerative disorders, and thus a shortened life-span.

Research in animal and human nutrition reveals that it is the subtle effects of imbalances, excesses, and deficiencies that matter in terms of long-term health. It is not within the scientific scope of nutritional science to declare the subtleties of these factors. There are more than forty essential nutrients known and more than fifty yet to be investigated in fresh foods. Science does not have 100% knowledge of anything, much less nutrition, so there are no universally accepted requirements for specific nutrients for birds, animals, or people. Nutrition is *not* an exact science. However, if we provide our birds with a variety of fresh foods, we can rest assured they are receiving a diet which will fulfill their dietary needs.

I often compare the diseases found in humans with the diseases found in animals and birds because in this context there is little difference between them. Humans, animals and birds all succumb to the same or similar degenerative diseases and illnesses from an unhealthy diet. They can similarly achieve vibrant health through nutritional and dietary methods.

It is fortuitous, that with time, increasing awareness abounds as to the importance of fresh raw or minimally cooked foods in our and our pets' diets. Many bird owners are feeding their birds more carefully and reading or defining the labels on food products to avoid potentially harmful chemical preservatives and additives. Research data is finally making it into mainstream literature which indicates the profound health benefits of fresh fruits and vegetables. The informed consumer now holds the key to providing their pets and themselves the *best* nutrition available.

As previously stated, there are no universally accepted requirements for specific nutrients for birds. Although all birds require the same nutrients, each species (or individual) may require more or less of a particular nutrient, such as one may require a higher or lower level of fat, protein, carbohydrate, vitamins, minerals, or water in their diet, and their caloric needs will vary. Energy foods are high in calories and are the main source of a bird's diet in the wild. However, in captivity with the lower activity level our bird's experience, the quantities of what we feed will depend on their lifestyles and the various stages (i.e., growth, molting, or breeding) they encounter throughout their lives. The amount of nutrients required by an individual bird is also influenced by its age, species, size, sex, environment, activity level, stress, illness/injury, hormonal status, nutritional status, and the type of diet consumed (its bioavailability). Additionally, because each bird is biochemically and genetically unique, with different strengths and weaknesses, their quantitative nutritional needs will differ.

Each nutrient has its own specific function, but no nutrient acts independent of another. All of the essential nutrients must be present in the diet in varying quantities over a period of days. It isn't necessary that your bird be served "complete nutrition" at every meal, every day. This is a fallacy indeed! A variety of healthy foods fed each day will add up to a properly balanced diet quite nicely.

Food processing, refining and soil nutrient depletion all play a part in vitamin/mineral deficiencies which result in symptoms and the illnesses associated with them. It should also be remembered, that while one bird may metabolize a nutrient sufficiently, another may not. We then have to determine why (such as a digestive disturbance), which can often be helped by an enzyme supplement, probiotics, and/or an improvement in diet. Sometimes just by adding a higher level of the particular nutrient(s) in question, we find that an improvement in health begins to take place.

Birds, with their high metabolic rate, require a diet rich in complex carbohydrates, such as whole grains, legumes, fruits and vegetables with their abundance of vitamins and minerals. Foods, which contain a high-water-content, such as raw fruits and vegetables are ideal for they are easily digested, provide our birds with enzymes, and other life-promoting elements. When selecting food for your birds, choose wholesome fresh, unrefined, *organic* foods and I believe, seventy percent of the food they eat should be water-rich foods.

Food enzymes, important in our bird's diet, are destroyed under low heat; between 105-118 degrees F, or slightly above a bird's body temperature. At all times, there are many types of enzymes working in their bodies. These work in blood, tissues,

3

organs and organ systems. For example, they maintain proper metabolic function of their bodies, stimulate production of antibodies that fight infection, and aid in the digestion of food. They are substances which make life possible. Vitamins, minerals, and hormones cannot do any work without the presence of enzymes, as they are responsible for all the body's biochemical reactions. Similarly, enzymes rely on vitamins/minerals (co-enzymes) for their proper function. A bird's digestive organs produce some enzymes to aid digestion; however, food (plant) enzymes are necessary for optimum health, therefore, fresh raw foods should form a large part of their diet. Whenever cooked foods are served, to promote maximum digestion and intestinal health, you can sprinkle a plant enzyme supplement over these foods.

Malabsorption of nutrients is a serious problem and its symptoms can include: weight loss, dry skin, feather loss, weakness, fatigue, and anemia. Those birds which suffer from this syndrome require more nutrients than others. In some cases, certain nutrients may need to be offered in a more easily assimilated form in older birds. These would include powders, liquids, or on occasion an injectable form, as advised by your avian veterinarian. Additional causes of the malfunction of absorption can be stress, over consumption of processed foods, refined sugars/carbohydrates, an enzyme deficient diet, an imbalance of the intestinal bacterial flora (candida), intestinal parasites, diarrhea and/or constipation, diseases of the pancreas, liver, and in turn result in digestive disorders. Under normal conditions, absorption is dependent on the body's needs; a bird who is deficient in a vitamin/mineral will absorb more of it than one who is sufficiently nourished.

Chapter 2
Avian Diets

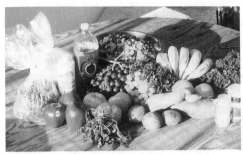

We are presently in an era where bird diets come in many forms. Some popular food items served are seeds, nuts, pellets, dried fruits and vegetables, fresh fruits and vegetables, sprouts, cooked beans and grains, pasta, and breads. We all know variety is the "spice of life" so some bird owners offer a combination or mixture of many of these items. While every bird owner has their favorite way to feed their birds, one thing we all have in common is the desire to provide the best possible diet for our birds.

When thinking about diet for our birds we want one that will (1) be relatively simple to prepare and serve, (2) be affordable, and (3) offer them the maximum opportunity to achieve optimum health. The diet dilemma begins...

These days many of us are concerned about how we can improve our bird's health and so we are questioning the quality and safety of the foods we serve them. When the discovery that an all seed diet was not providing our birds with all of their nutritional needs, many commercial diets were developed and sold as "complete nutrition". However, nutritional science is an inexact science and so a commercial feed can never be "complete" in terms of what any of our pets need. Our pets are all biochemically and genetically unique, therefore nutritional requirements will vary. The "everything your bird needs in a bag" concept is simply marketing hype.

We have also been mislead by the many attractive commercial advertisements which display whole grains, vegetables, and fruits; however, what you see may not always be what you get. There are virtually no whole ingredients in a highly processed commercial feed. Your pet is merely consuming fractionated ingredients from the original whole foods source, along with synthetic nutrients. Isolated, synthetic vitamins, minerals, amino acids and so forth must be added to these products before packaging, because many of the nutrients have been diminished by the processing procedures or were simply not there to begin with. These products provide the minimum level of nutrients for the "average" bird's needs and are sold as "complete and balanced". We all know that none of our birds are "average" and so this disregards each bird's biochemical individuality and leaves open the chance for nutrient excesses or deficiencies which can eventually lead to illness and disease. Few long-term studies on bird food have been conducted and few if any generational trials have been conducted. No one knows what the 100% perfect level of nutrients are, so feeding trials and feed analysis cannot assure that a food is sufficiently balanced for the widely differing biochemical individuality of each bird. The manufacturer of a product conducts the feeding trials and therefore the trial results are not always flawless, scientific, or unbiased.

As a result of the alluring and convincing marketing skills of the many bird food companies, many bird owners have sadly come to rely increasingly on processed convenience foods (similar to the cat and dog bagged diets) and consider them to be the best way to provide their birds with the proper nutrients. With good intentions, many bird owners purchase these products based on hearsay and the substantial claims made of the products' complete nutrition, with little to no knowledge of the foods composition and value. To be an educated consumer for our birds, as well as for ourselves, requires that we take the time to research the safety and quality of each ingredient on the label *before* we serve it to our pets. A Consumer's Dictionary to Food Additives by Ruth Winter is highly recommended to aid in this research. For free literature about pet food manufacturing contact the Animal Protection Institute of America (800)-348-7387.

While some people may feel that if a bird is eating a processed, fabricated diet that contains all "known" nutrients, it is complete and all that is needed; my opinion differs. While some of these products might provide some health benefits if they were free of artificial additives and made-up of high quality ingredients; in terms of a healthful daily diet, I don't believe they are adequate substitutes for the nutrients found in whole, fresh foods. Pellets are a very "unnatural" food and a questionable source of nutrition for our birds. If a parrot stumbled upon them in the wild it would not even consider them edible unless it was starving, there was a food shortage, or there was nothing else available to eat. (Unfortunately, in captivity many breeders in their zest to do the right thing, are weaning their babies onto pellets and the birds imprint on these foods

6

and unknowingly think they are natural—the same as cats, dogs, ferrets, and other companion animals.)

A heat-treated synthetic feed is generally more difficult to digest and therefore less bioavailable to the body and some important food elements may even be transformed into toxins and carcinogens by the chemical reactions of the heating process. The guaranteed percentage of crude protein and fat listed on the label means very little, because the crude nutrient content does not accurately reflect the degree of nutrient bioavailability, nor does the chemical analysis always reflect the exact level of nutrients. The pretty colors and cute little shapes of these foods are all achieved during the harsh processing techniques used in the pet food factories to appeal to the buyers of these products. In a nutshell, pellets were designed for profit volume, not optimum health.

Dangers of the nutritionally complete concept:

1) Ignores individuality. This should give you greater insight into why some birds may do well on one diet and poorly on another. Some birds will require more or less of a particular nutrient.

2) We don't have complete knowledge of what our birds require, therefore how can a manufacturer claim with any certainty that its products are nutritionally complete.

3) Processing can decrease nutrient content and bioavailability and create new toxic compounds that are potentially carcinogenic and free radical generating.

4) False sense of security -- the nutritionally complete claim gives consumers a false impression that regulators can guarantee quality. They cannot!

There are really no similarities between a synthetic pelleted feed and a varied natural whole foods diet. Simply put: One diet is artificially man-made (dead) and the other nature-made (alive). Many of the commercial diets contain chemical dyes, chemical preservatives to extend shelf-life (i.e., Ethoxyquin, BHT, and/or BHA), refined sugar (sucrose, corn syrup) and other non-nutrient additives, which I believe sooner or later will have a negative impact on the health of our birds, causing digestive tract disorders, immune system disorders, behavioral disorders, feather and skin problems, a variety of degenerative diseases and organ damage.

Not only are commercial food products primarily made-up of fragmented substances and isolated, synthetic vitamins and minerals, most do not contain important elements like enzymes, chlorophyll, and other natural beneficial substances which are found in natural foods. For quite awhile now, it has been recognized that fresh natural foods contain many more substances than just vitamins, minerals, and other healthful, energy promoting foods, i.e., natural antioxidant compounds: carotenoids, phytochemicals, and the polyphenols. These substances (nutraceuticals) are all biologically active components of plant life and possess natural disease resistance properties for the plants themselves as well as those who eat them.

Scientists are discovering more new substances all the time in fruits, vegetables, grains, legumes, and seeds. These substances are often found to be beneficial to our health, such as by blocking the steps which lead to cancer formation. Nutraceuticals have also been shown to boost the immune system, stimulate the production of enzymes in the body for effective digestion and detoxification, possess antibiotic and antioxidant properties, and many other healing qualities. So the more that is learned about these beneficial elements in fresh foods the more it becomes evident that these elements would collectively play a major role in keeping both human and animal bodies healthy and ultimately disease-free. There isn't a commercial food product or nutritional supplement available that can provide our birds with the outstanding goodness that is to be found in Mother Nature's garden.

By adding fresh foods to a commercial diet we are improving upon them (though many commercial feed companies will warn you not to add a substantial amount of fresh foods to their diet because you may upset the delicate nutritional balance of the pelleted feed -- marketing hype again!). Fresh foods added to a pelleted diet can only enhance it! However, if we feed a well-balanced variety of natural, fresh foods each day, then it is not necessary to also serve a pelleted feed. The complexity of nutritive components in fresh foods can provide our pets with the nourishment to support their health -- as nature intended.

Birds in the wild do not always receive all the essential nutrients every day, but may receive them over a period of days. This "pounding" of all the essential known nutrients into our birds' bodies each day with a synthetic diet is what can cause overdoses (hypervitaminosis) and organ damage. On the contrary, if a feed is inadequate in a particular nutrient(s) or is insufficiently digested, it can cause under doses (hypovitaminosis) and malnutrition. It is very difficult to overdose on nutrients with a *natural* feed. If a large *variety* of fresh foods are served each day this will more than adequately provide our birds with all the nutrients needed for long-term optimum health.

Manufacturers often use scare tactics to persuade the unknowledgable consumer to buy their feed. They claim that they are the only ones that *know* what we should be feeding our animals, or tell us that a bagged diet is vastly superior over a naturally grown diet. Nonsense! Sadly, the public at large has been so conditioned and shamed by this information from the bird food companies, that they are afraid to trust their own instincts as to what *is* a healthy diet for their birds. While it may be helpful, we *do not* all require a degree in nutrition to provide ourselves, our family, and our pets a healthy diet. A basic knowledge and understanding of foods, their nutritional value, and a little common sense goes a long way.

I think of my flock as if they were my children. So if my pediatrician were to recommend a bag of dry food, and tell me that this is the only thing I'll ever need to feed my children for the rest of their life, and that *nothing* I could prepare was better, or even adequate... you guessed it, I'd look for another doctor! Certainly our children *and* our birds deserve more than just kibble out of can or bag. I often pose the following questions to people who are on the edge of trying to make a decision on whether to feed their birds pellets. Would you want to eat them? Would you serve them to your children and other loved ones? If not, then *don't* serve them to your pets.

Chapter 3
A Naturally Healthy Diet.

Foods are healthiest as close to nature and as unprocessed as possible. Serving our birds wholesome foods is not much different from feeding ourselves a healthy diet. Mixing grains and legumes creates a high quality protein meal; nuts and seeds provide an excellent source of protein, some vitamins, minerals, and the essential fatty acids. The chief contributions that fruits provide are beta carotene, vitamin C and some minerals. Vegetables offer our birds nearly all of the vitamins and minerals required for good health and can supply significant protein, with little, to no, fat. Most vegetables contain some of the essential amino acids with many containing them all. If you feed fruits, vegetables, legumes, grains, nuts, seeds and sprouts on a regular basis, your bird is receiving all the amino acids necessary for a healthy body. It was once commonly believed that a great deal of effort was needed to "balance" the vegetable proteins to form "complete" protein. Most scientists realize now that a diversified vegetable diet will supply adequate protein for our health needs. Vegetables, legumes, grains, nuts and seeds contain more than enough protein for the growth and maintenance of your bird's body. It would be nearly impossible for your bird to develop a protein deficiency if it is eating a variety of plant foods. Plant foods also provide those very important substances described earlier: Nutraceuticals.

Do it yourself! Preparing a fresh diet, consisting of wholesome ingredients, need not require a tremendous amount of time and preparation. In fact, with the "mash" diet, preparation is done in advance at your convenience. This method of feeding eliminates the daily slicing and dicing of fruits and vegetables. I make up ten days worth for nearly twenty pair of birds; which takes about one and a half hours to complete. (Less time for fewer birds.) Then, serving is as simple as scooping out the correct amount for each bird or pair.

Have you ever wondered how much of what you were serving your birds was actually eaten? How many times have you found most of their food thrown about, picked at, and wasted on the ground or at the bottom of their cages? We all know birds don't have good manners at meal time and you never really know if they are getting all of the nutrients necessary for proper health. Well, the mash diet should help alleviate any doubts as all ingredients are minced through a food processor with the idea being that your birds cannot select only a few favorite items, but will receive a wide range of nutrients with every beakful.

To begin, all ingredients are placed through the food processor *briefly* (with the exception of certain foods eaten readily), and then scooped into a 20 quart stainless steel pot for mixing. (Note: Remember to always place cover over the pot in between adding an ingredient to prevent oxidation from exposure to air.) The mash is then placed in air tight containers and stored in the freezer, but must be removed to the refrigerator for thawing well in advance (30 to 36 hours for a five cup container). Scheduled feeding times are at 8:00 am (mash) and 2:00 p.m. (seed mixture), simulating the natural eating patterns of birds in the wild. The 8:00 a.m. feeding provides them with enough to fill their crops throughout the morning hours. Although each pair is treated individually, about 1/2 cup per pair is the average (for medium-sized parrots). As you learn how much each bird or pair will eat in each time period the amount can be adjusted so that none is wasted. Any uneaten mash should be discarded after four to six hours to prevent spoilage, which if eaten, could cause a bacterial infection. Special care should be taken in this matter, particularly in the warmer months. These frequent feeding times will also allow you the opportunity to observe your birds often, which is very important in keeping you closely in tune to their overall health. Feeding times may vary and are adjusted to your schedule; these are guidelines only.

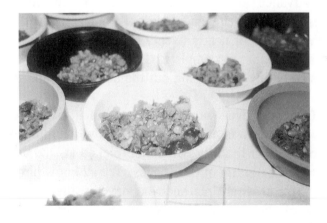

MASH INGREDIENTS: (for twenty pair)

Frozen organic vegetables - (corn, green beans, carrots, peas) 12 lb.

Fresh organic vegetables - 1 lb. parsley, 5 large tomatoes, 3 chayote (fed raw), 3 medium sweet potatoes or yams, 4 medium white potatoes (fed lightly steamed, skins included).

Bean mix - 1/2 cup each of the following beans and peas: black-eyed peas, pinto beans, kidney beans, adzuki beans, green and yellow split peas, garbanzo beans, black beans, soy beans, mung beans. (Rinse and drain well, soak in cold water 6 to 8 hours in refrigerator.) After soaking boil for 10 minutes, simmer for 20 minutes, using only enough water so that none remains after cooking, (to preserve valuable vitamins).

Grains - 1/2 cup each,: wheat berry, pearl barley, triticale, brown rice. Add to beans, soak, and boil.

Organic greens - (fresh grown) comfrey and/or mustard greens. Comfrey, (an herb) which provides vitamin A, B-complex, C, & E. Up to 33% protein is contained in the leaves and it is high in minerals. Mustard greens are high in vitamins A, B, C, calcium and iron. Frilly-leafed and broad leafed are available. (About 1 dozen large leaves are used.)

Organic Fruit - 5 large bananas, 5 large apples, 1 1/2 lbs. of grapes fed whole, (1/4 cup strawberries or cranberries seasonally.)

Seeds - 1/4 cup each: pumpkin seeds and sesame seeds. Both provide calcium along with zinc, which aids in fertility. Sesame seeds also provide an additional source of 8 "essential" amino acids which cannot be manufactured by a parrot's body.

Vitamin and mineral supplements - 1/4 cup powered kelp (contains iodine, therefore helps to prevent thyroid disorders, such as goiter), 1/4 cup blue green algae or alfalfa powder (aids in digestion, strengthens immune system, and is nutrient-dense).

Mash Formula Breakdown -- 10 days worth!

Ingredients	For 1 Medium sized parrot	For 10 Pair	For 20 Pair
Frozen Organic Vegetables	1/3 pound	6 pounds	12 pounds
Fresh Organic Vegetables			
parsley	1/2 ounce	1/2 pound	1 pound
large tomatoes	1/8 large tomato	2.5	5
chayote	1/2 ounce	1.5	3
medium sweet potatoes/yams	3/4 ounce	1.3	3
medium white potatoes	3/4 ounce	2	4
Bean Mix			
black-eyed peas	1/2 teaspoon	1/4 cup	1/2 cup
pinto beans	1/2 teaspoon	1/4 cup	1/2 cup
kidney beans	1/2 teaspoon	1/4 cup	1/2 cup
adzuki or mung beans	1/2 teaspoon	1/4 cup	1/2 cup
green split peas	1/2 teaspoon	1/4 cup	1/2 cup
yellow split peas	1/2 teaspoon	1/4 cup	1/2 cup
garbanzo beans	1/2 teaspoon	1/4 cup	1/2 cup
black beans	1/2 teaspoon	1/4 cup	1/2 cup
soy beans	1/2 teaspoon	1/4 cup	1/2 cup
Grains			
wheat berry	1/2 teaspoon	1/4 cup	1/2 cup
pearl barley	1/2 teaspoon	1/4 cup	1/2 cup
triticale	1/2 teaspoon	1/4 cup	1/2 cup
brown rice	1/2 teaspoon	1/4 cup	1/2 cup
Organic Greens			
comfrey and/or mustard greens	1/3 large leaf	6 large leaves	12 large leaves
Organic Fruit			
large bananas	1/8 banana	2 1/2	5
large apples	1/8 apple	2 1/2	5
whole grapes	1/2 ounce	3/4 pound	1.5 pounds
strawberries or cranberries seasonally	1/4 teaspoon	2 tbspns	1/4 cup
Seeds			
pumpkin/sesame seeds	1/4 teaspoon	2 tbspns	1/4 cup
Vitamins/Minerals			
powdered kelp	1/4 teaspoon	2 tbspns	1/4 cup
blue green algae or alfalfa powder	1/4 teaspoon	2 tbspns	1/4 cup

This recipe can be used as a guide for a healthy diet. You may substitute an item for another equivalent food item; for instance, if a particular one is seasonally unavailable. Examples: Collard or dandelion greens in place of comfrey or zucchini in place of chayote. In addition to the mash diet, orange chunks, celery sticks, and almonds are served regularly as well. Also, occasionally served is mashed hard-boiled egg with shell included (boiled 20 minutes), whole grain wheat bread, and a natural cornbread, which is always eagerly consumed.

Supplements.

The high phosphorus to calcium ratio in most foods requires an increase in calcium through a quality supplement. The ratio of calcium to phosphorus, should be 2.5:1, including D3. Extra calcium is provided daily by the use of a **calcium magnesium liquid** for the requirements of the African Greys, while other species receive it regularly with frequency depending upon age, activity level, and breeding cycles. Juvenile birds (under 1 year) and pairs which are aging or less active receive it more often, as are birds prior to and during egg laying, and while raising young. Remember that birds under stress (which includes extreme heat or cold) need additional calcium, as well as an increase in all essential nutrients. We add 1 tsp. of the Calcium Magnesium Liquid daily to the mash for each pair of Greys; other medium-sized birds, e.g., Amazons and Pionus, 1/2 tsp. per pair. Small birds, such as cockatiel size, 1/4 tsp. per pair. Large parrots, same as for Greys. Reduce amount for a single bird.

An aged garlic extract can be sprinkled over the mash daily for its benefits in aiding digestion, stimulating the immune system, and keeping your birds resistant to infection and disease. We use *apple cider* **vinegar** (ACV) over the mash using a plastic squirt bottle; 1/2 tsp. for medium to large size birds, 1/4 tsp. for smaller species. ACV is an immunity enhancer; its natural antibiotic action protects your birds from infections. It is rich in enzymes, potassium, and other important minerals, and aids in digestion and the assimilation of food. An organic non-distilled brand is recommended.

The **seeds, nuts, and grains** which are offered in the afternoon, make-up about 30% of their diet. Most seeds are beneficial, but you must be sure they come from a quality source. Ideally, some can be grown in your own environment, if space permits. The basis of our raw organic seed mixture is hulled millet 80%, hulled sunflower 5%, shelled peanuts 5%, rolled oats 5%, and buckwheat 5%. The most important nutritive elements of seeds are the B-complex vitamins, vitamins A and E, unsaturated fatty acids, protein, phosphorous, and calcium. For example, pumpkin seeds, sesame seeds, and sunflower seeds are high in protein, plus all of the above vitamins as well as magnesium, zinc, iodine, and potassium.

The value of seeds, nuts, and grains along with beans and peas, are unsurpassed, especially in the sprouted form. Sprouting seeds will increase their total vitamin content and may be added to the morning mash. Seeds also have a positive effect on birds by supplying quick energy, beak stimulation, and are certainly healthful in rationed amounts. Over indulgence of seed, especially fatty seed, such as sunflower, peanut, etc., may crowd out other essential foods from the diet and can therefore result in nutritional deficiency as well as obesity. Your seed mix should be stored in a cool, dry place, away from direct light, and in air-tight containers to prevent rancidity caused by oxidation. Some protection from rancidity will be provided by vitamin E which is a natural antioxidant, and present in varying amounts in oil-bearing foods. No more than six weeks worth should be purchased in advance.

Wild birds can also benefit from organically-grown seeds along with the other foods they find in their wild habitat. Pesticide-free seeds will help to promote the health, reproduction, and increase the longevity of all of the birds in your life.

Food Storage and Cooking Methods:

Purchasing fresh foods and keeping them that way isn't always an easy task. Fruits and vegetables, once harvested, begin to immediately lose their value from exposure to light, warmth and air. Transportation from the field to the market also diminishes some nutrients. In addition, the time the fresh food sits on the shelf at the market and in your home will promote losses. Overripe fruits and vegetables contain less nutrients and enzymes than fresh fruits and vegetables. Fresh groceries should be purchased frequently and foods should be eaten shortly after purchase for their maximum nutrient content. Store fresh produce in moisture-free refrigerator bins; maintain temperature between 32-35 degrees F.

There are certain foods which require cooking for their maximum digestibility and to eliminate natural toxins, such as grains, legumes and some root vegetables. Cooking of any kind will breakdown some nutrients, but make others more bioavailable. I recommend only cooking what really needs to be cooked and serving most vegetables raw. There are nutrient-saving cooking methods which will be health-promoting for your birds. These methods include steaming, parboiling, crock-pot or pressure cooking. But as a rule, the least amount of cooking the better, with a higher level of nutrients retained as a result. If fresh vegetables are unavailable, use frozen versus canned, as they contain more nutritional value. Frozen foods should be prepared and served as soon as possible after thawing.

Handfeeding Formula.

The recipe below is based on the adult mash diet listed in this chapter. It is the formula I feed my babies. I add a probiotic supplement to their morning feeding during the first few weeks of life. Other supplements which may be added are liquid or powdered garlic, echinacea, and vitamin C. You can modify this recipe for feeding only one bird.

HANDFEEDING FORMULA.

2 cups "mash"
1/2 cup cultured buttermilk
1/2 cup peanut butter (fresh-made, certified organic)
1/3 cup sesame oil (cold-pressed)
2 tbs. calcium magnesium liquid
1/2 cup filtered water
✱All ingredients are placed in the blender and pureed

This formula texture is thick, which is fine for older chicks. Dilute it with more filtered water to feed day one chicks (very thin, broth-like), gradually reducing the water as the babies grow older. Store in airtight containers in the freezer and thaw daily portions in advance. We never heat the formula any higher than the low side of a chick's body temperature, which on average is 107 F. to assure the formula is at the proper temperature for feeding (104-106 F.) This retains more of the nutrients. Never boil as cooking destroys the enzymes. Spoon feeding is our method of choice for our babies, as we feel it is a more natural feeling for the bird to pump for its food, as it would when parent-fed.

Alicia's Au Naturel' Cornbread Recipe:

For conditioning, breeding, and weaning birds, this cornbread is nutritional, and thoroughly enjoyed.

CORNBREAD RECIPE

1 cup whole wheat flour
2 tbs. Sucanat®
1 tbs. baking powder (non-aluminum)
1/2 tsp. (kelp or dulse)
1 cup cornmeal
2 eggs, beaten
1/4 cup vegetable oil
1 cup milk
1 tbs. soybean isolate
1 tbs. nutritional yeast
1/4 cup raw wheat germ

Preheat oven to 325 degrees. Melt butter in a 8"x8"x2" Pyrex pan. Mix all ingredients in a medium bowl, and bake for 25 minutes. It may be cut into squares and frozen, to be thawed for future use.

CANARIES: as the birds begin to fledge and eat on their own they are provided with the cornbread as needed (as well as seed, fruit, and greens) until they are able to crack seed and have completed their baby molt. It may also be given as a healthy treat throughout the year.

FINCHES: enjoyed primarily during the feeding and raising of young.

HOOKBILLS: it encourages breeding, it can be added to the soft food that the parent birds feed to their offspring, and as a weaning food when they begin to eat independently. Also enjoyed as a healthy treat throughout the year.

Chapter 4
Anti-Nutritional and Toxic Compounds in Foods.

Plant foods are composed of a large number of chemical compounds. Toxicity may result from the consumption of a plant or plant part that contains a high level of a toxic substance. Cooking reduces the toxicity of many of the plant foods listed below.

Enzyme inhibitors are proteins found in raw beans, but they also occur in grains, seeds, nuts, potatoes, eggplant and onions. They restrict digestion of these foods causing the pancreas to increase its output of digestive enzymes. Cooking may neutralize the inhibitors in these foods but kills the needed digestive enzymes inherent in the food. Sprouting beans and grains are better alternatives than cooking them. The enzyme inhibitors have been "dismantled" during the growing process leaving the enzymes free to digest the food.

All beans, some grains, and potatoes, in the raw form, contain a toxin called **lectins**. Lectins are carbohydrate-binding proteins, that cause agglutination of red blood cells, and may affect the intestines and prevent absorption of nutrients. Boiling beans, grains, and potatoes for 10 minutes, before simmering, destroys these lectins. Certain varieties of lima beans contain **cyanogenic glycosides**. The boiling of these beans (in an uncovered pot) releases the hydrogen cyanide gases and renders them safe if fed in moderation.

I am often asked if parsley is poisonous to birds. It is not. However, certain plants, such as parsley, parsnip and carrot leaves, celery... have the ability to cause a photosensitivity reaction if an individual is exposed to excessive sunlight after ingestion. Those plants containing **furocoumarins**, including psoralens, are classified as phototoxic. Phototoxic reactions occur by the activation of furocoumarins by photons, resulting in free radical damage, such as cell damage, erythema, or bulla formation. Again, this photosensitivity would only occur in response to exposure of excessive solar radiation after the ingestion of a sensitizing food. So parsley served in moderation is a healthy food for birds. Along with its high content of beta carotene, it contains many other useful vitamins and minerals.

Cruciferous vegetables -- broccoli, brussel sprouts, cabbage, kale, mustard greens, turnip, watercress and other species of the genus Brassica are known to contain chemical compounds called

goitrogenic glycosides or **glucosinolates**. These glycosides can damage thyroid function and cause goiter by preventing the uptake of iodine and limiting thyroxine production. Glycosides are responsible for the sharp taste of some members of this genus. While these chemicals are present in all parts of the plant, the highest concentration is known to be in the seeds. This is Nature's own defense system; a protection from insects and other pests. These chemicals are a natural protection, generally in micro amounts, and considered harmless if consumed in small quantities as a part of a balanced diet. However, feeding foods of the genus Brassica could pose a particular concern if a bird has a thyroid disorder or if these foods are consumed in large amounts. Cooking these vegetables will destroy the glycosides. While I advocate feeding raw foods whenever possible for the optimum health benefits, if fed raw, smaller amounts can be served.

There is ongoing research into the many beneficial chemical compounds found in members of the Brassica family. These vegetables have been recognized for their ability to stimulate the immune system, and act as an antidote in cancer prevention. They contain an abundance of nutrients -- vitamins, minerals, trace minerals, amino acids, essential fatty acids, and other natural chemicals, such as sulforaphane (in broccoli), which may inhibit illness and disease.

Oxalic acid is a compound found in beet greens, spinach, kale, soybeans, almonds, rhubarb, and to a lesser extent buckwheat, carrots, parsley, and string beans, which can inhibit the absorption of calcium and other minerals in the intestines. Oxalic acid is the waste product of plant metabolism and is found in practically all plant families, usually in highest concentrations in older plants. Along with the plant's age, the oxalate content varies with seasonal, climatic, and soil conditions. Rhubarb, beets, and spinach are among the highest in oxalate content, though still considered in safe levels. If large amounts of oxalate-containing foods were consumed, the oxalates may combine with free calcium in the digestive tract to form insoluble calcium oxalate. This could result in a calcium deficiency (hypocalcemia - a low level of blood calcium), particularly if the diet is already low in calcium. Additionally, insoluble calcium oxalate crystals may be deposited in the kidneys and other organs thus causing mechanical damage. Under normal circumstances, oxalates in moderate amounts are broken down by the bacteria in the bird's digestive tract after they've done their job of promoting digestion. In general, a healthy bird receiving a well-balanced varied diet will never have a problem with oxalate-containing foods.

The white potato, tomatoes, eggplant, and peppers are members of the Nightshade family. These veggies contain varying concentrations of solanine. Solanine is a poisonous chemical called a **glycoalkaloid**. Potatoes normally contain harmless quantities of solanine, it is only when exposed to light or extreme temperature that they develop larger amounts. It is generally recognized that the parts of the potato which carries the potential to be toxic are the eyes, sprouts, and berries, as these parts contain the highest concentration of toxins. Unripe, green, or spoiled potatoes are also potentially very dangerous. Livestock have been poisoned from eating green, decayed, or sprouting potatoes. However, most cases of potato poisoning result from eating potatoes which are green (chlorophyll) from having been grown close to the surface or stored improperly after harvesting, i.e., exposure to light/heat and/or have sprouted. As a result the alkaloid content may increase to toxic levels. Boiling in water reduces the alkaloid content from green or sprouted potatoes, but does not eliminate them. If potatoes become green they can be stored in darkness for about two weeks. They should be eaten only after all green has disappeared, or you can cut away and remove all parts that are green (always remove the eyes and sprouts.) Avoiding green potatoes to begin with is your best option. Remember to store potatoes in a cool, dry dark location. Additionally, an infection with potato blight disease fungus increases the toxin concentration.

Members of the Nightshade family can pose a health threat to those with arthritic conditions, such as gout. The alkaloids in these vegetables may increase joint pain. Some (human) individuals are allergic to them and are affected considerably by their consumption. The alkaloids in the nightshades may also disturb calcium metabolism, therefore these veggies should be consumed in a diet where calcium-rich foods are provided. Only the stems and leaves of tomatoes are toxic. The leaves, unripe and overripe fruits of eggplant are toxic.

I believe we can safely feed potatoes and other members of the Nightshade family to our birds if they are selected, stored, and prepared properly. Interestingly, research shows that raw potatoes contain protease inhibitors which are anti-cancer compounds and known to block carcinogens. The chemicals in potatoes may prevent viruses. Researchers have also found the potato skin is particularly healthy in regard to preventing cell mutations which are the precursor to cancer. While some plants are indeed toxic, many plants are used for medicinal purposes as well as for their nutritive value.

➡The following foods and other substances have been known to be toxic to birds at low levels of concentration or are simply unhealthy and should be avoided!

refined sugar
refined white-flour
soda pop
alcohol
avocado
caffeine
chocolate
dairy products
salt
fried foods
chemical preservatives
chemical dyes
artificial flavoring

Chapter 5
*Macro*nutrients and *Micro*nutrients.

Macronutrients:

Macronutrients provide energy and aid in the maintenance and repair of the body. Their ability is expressed in **calories**, the amount of chemical energy that is released as heat when food is metabolized.

Carbohydrates include sugars, starches and fiber. Sugars and starches help maintain the glucose level. Carbohydrates are the most efficient fuel for the body because they can be broken down quickly, especially those from fruit. Starches require a longer time for enzymes to break down their polysaccharides parts to simple sugars and then to glucose for absorption. The glucose is used by the tissues of the brain, nervous system, and muscles. The rest is stored as glycogen in the liver, muscles, skin, and throughout the body. Carbohydrates also help to regulate protein and fat metabolism.

Refined carbohydrates should be avoided as they are empty calories and provide no nutritional value. Fructose, such as is found in fruits are a simple carbohydrate composed of easily digestible monosaccharides. Maltose, such as is found in sprouting seeds are composed of disaccharides which require some digestion. Complex carbohydrates or polysaccharides, such as grains, legumes and vegetables require a longer time for digestion and contain a lot of nutritional extras--vitamins and minerals and often appreciable amounts of water and fiber. Raw fruits and vegetables are excellent for weight reduction for those parrots who could afford to lose a few grams, such as some individuals of the Amazon and Pionus genus. Weight loss can be achieved by regulating the amount of calories consumed versus the energy expenditure of your bird. In other words, if the calories in their food total to more than what can be burned off by the basal metabolism, physical activity, and diet induced thermogenesis (i.e., digestion, absorption, etc.), then weight gain will likely occur. In this case, reducing the caloric amount offered will help trim down an overweight bird. In addition, excessive fat intake will cause abnormally slow digestion and absorption, resulting in maldigestion.

Cellulose, also known as fiber, is found in the skins of fruits and vegetables and helps to maintain normal intestinal function. Birds do not possess the enzyme cellulase and therefore can not digest cellulose by their intestinal tract. Plant foods eaten raw contain cellulase and will help aid in the break down of cellulose. Hemicellulose, found in the cell walls of plant food, is related to cellulose. The bacteria in the intestines can help break down hemicellulose. Lignin and pectin are two other forms of fiber.

Proteins are essential for the health and maintenance of the body's tissues, growth, development, reproduction, and resistance to infection. During digestion, protein is broken down into simpler units called amino acids or polypeptides. Protein is more plentiful than any other substance in your bird's body. It is essential to good health and is the major source of building material for feathers, skin, nails, muscles, blood, all internal organs and function as enzymes, antibodies, hemoglobin, genes, and hormones. Feathers are primarily made up of keratin: a fibrous protein substance. Beaks, which are made from bone, nails, and leg scales are also made up of keratin. Collagen, another important fibrous protein, forms the material for bones, ligaments, tendons, cartilage and connective tissue. Elastin, which is very similar to collagen, is a protein constituting the basic substance of elastic tissue.

Protein is also a source for heat and energy. When enough fats and carbohydrates are utilized or, excess protein is consumed, this energy is saved and is converted by the liver and stored as fat in the body tissues for later use. A bird's body requires approximately 22 plus amino acids in specific patterns to make protein. Amino acids synthesize complete proteins and are the units from which protein is constructed. All but ten of these amino acids can be produced in the body by the liver. These ten must be supplied in the diet and are termed essential amino acids. They are: methionine, threonine, leucine, lysine, tryptophan, valine, isoleucine, phenylalanine and (histidine and arginine) are essential during the rapid growth phase of young birds.

It is not necessary for each meal to contain a complete protein. The liver stores the essential amino acids for a short period of time and releases them into the bloodstream as needed for building cells, enzymes, and hormones. The liver acts as a buffer in the event that an excess amount of protein is consumed. When there is a high amino acid concentration in the blood, a large proportion of the amino acids are absorbed by the liver cells and converted into small proteins, while some amino acids will be excreted via the kidneys in the form of uric acid. On the other hand, when there is a deficiency of certain amino acids, the liver, as well as other body cells, will release the missing amino acids, if it has them in storage.

When an illness or trauma (stress) occurs, an increase in protein is necessary in order to assist in the healing process. When a food contains all the essential amino acids it is called a complete protein. A food that is low in, or lacks an essential amino acid it is called an incomplete protein. Some vegetables, beans, and grains are incomplete, but combined provide an excellent source of complete protein and can provide all the protein your bird's body requires. For example, legumes are rich in lysine, but low in methionine. Grains are rich in methionine, but low in lysine. So when you combine these foods they compliment one another and create a complete protein. Soy beans, lentils, sunflower, sesame, and peanuts are a complete protein. When feeding a varied fresh diet, concern about protein complimentarity is not necessary. A diverse plant food diet will provide more than enough protein to meet the needs of your pet bird. Carbohydrates and fats help protein to be utilized efficiently and supports growth. An inadequate supply of protein will cause stunted growth, feather and joint deformities, and weakening muscles in youngsters, and in adults, loss of energy, depression, and a greater susceptibility to infection. However, a diet too high in protein may encourage calcium excretion, deplete minerals from bones, liver dysfunction, kidney failure, or gout. Yogurt, green leafy vegetables, and soybeans are all good sources of both protein and calcium.

Fats (lipids) There are three classes of lipids: triglycerides, phospholipids, and sterols. All fats are composed of either saturated or unsaturated fatty acids. Most plant foods and fish are unsaturated and animal foods are saturated, mono unsaturated or poly-unsaturated. These fats provide a concentrated energy source, insulate the body and are necessary for the utilization of the fat-soluble vitamins (A, D, E, & K). Lipids work with other nutrients to support the structure and function of every cell, aid in the absorption of vitamin D for proper calcium metabolism and assist in normal reproduction function. Fats are stored in the liver in the form of glycogen. When needed, enzymes breakdown the glycogen to glucose which provides energy. Fat is also stored in muscle under the skin and throughout the body. The diet must be composed of sufficient amounts, and void of any excess which may be harmful to your bird's health.

The three important essential unsaturated fatty acids (EFA's), are linoleic, linolenic and arachidonic acids. These fatty acids cannot be made by the body. Arachidonic and linolenic acids can be synthesized from linoleic acid if it is supplied in sufficient amounts in the diet. Fatty acids are best absorbed in the presence of vitamin E. Seeds/nuts are excellent sources of vitamin E, plus a mixed balance of linolenic acid and linoleic acid. They should be fed as a part of an overall balanced diet, which includes lots of fresh vegetables and fruits.

The amount of linoleic acid needed for health varies with climate, levels of stress, activity level, nutritional status, and individual differences. Linoleic acid, independently, has no biological activity, but must be converted in the body to those fatty acids which are active. Linoleic acid is the precursor to the prostaglandins -- a family of hormone-like compounds that control every cell and organ of the body. If an essential fatty acid deficiency is suspected, nutritional supplements such as flax (oil or meal), fish oil and evening primrose oil can be added to your bird's diet.

EFA's help keep your bird's feathers and skin healthy by preventing dryness, itchiness, allergies, and feather loss. They also regulate normal glandular activity of the adrenal and thyroid glands, are necessary for normal growth, and healthy blood and nerves. Additionally, they strengthen the immune system and have been indicated to have anti-cancer properties, and may be therapeutic for heart disease, high cholesterol, arthritis, gout, and respiratory disorders.

Micronutrients:

Vitamins (organic substances) and minerals (inorganic substances) work together synergistically and are essential to maintaining health and fighting disease. There are various vitamins and minerals which have been found to be essential for achieving optimum health and most of them cannot be synthesized by a bird's body.

VITAMINS: Vitamins are organic compounds which are required in very small amounts. Water-soluble vitamins are B and C; the fat soluble are A, D, E, & K. Fat soluble vitamins require dietary fats and the secretion of bile acids for efficient absorption. Fats are stored in the liver or fat tissue for long periods of time whereas water-soluble vitamins are stored briefly, leaving the kidney through the ureters in the form of urine and are later excreted from the cloaca. Vitamins regulate the chemical processes of the body, and are essential for the growth development and maintenance of good health. Minerals assist with this, and in the formation of new tissue, including bones, blood, and in the regulation of water. Both are important in the function of enzyme systems.

—**Vitamin A.** Retinol (preformed; ready for the body to use immediately and found in animal foods) and/or beta carotene/provitamin A (precursor to vitamin A and found in the fat-soluble pigments of many types of plant food) are required for a healthy immune system and resistance to infection. Vitamin A functions as an antioxidant by protecting against damage to cell membranes caused by "free radicals" in the environment. It is also essential for the health of the eyes, feathers, epithelial tissue (i.e., lungs, skin, and intestines), growth and bone formation, reproduction, and may prevent liver disorders, cancer and other diseases.

Although overdoses of certain fat soluble forms of vitamin A could cause toxicity, it is generally regarded as safe. However, beta-carotene may not be properly converted to vitamin A by those with diabetes, hypothyroidism or liver dysfunction. A natural alternative: vitamin A and D from emulsified (unfortified) cod liver oil (naturally flavored) -- we use 1 tbs. per lb. of seed mix.

Vitamin A in the synthetic form (palmitate or acetate) is generally water-soluble for quick absorption and can be toxic if offered at high levels. Symptoms of vitamin A toxicity or hypervitaminosis A may include loss of appetite, feather loss, diarrhea, skin scaling, itchiness, lethargy, weight loss, or enlargement of the liver and spleen, bone disease, or kidney failure. Cold weather, infection, cortisone, excess iron and sugar may deplete vitamin A from the body. A deficiency of vitamin A may lead to appetite loss, allergies, dry feathers and skin, follicular hyperkeratosis, feather loss, sinusitis, and susceptibility to bacterial, viral and yeast infection. Dietary sources of retinol may be found in egg yolk, cheese, and cod liver oil. Dietary sources of carotene are found chiefly in richly colored orange, yellow and green fruits and vegetables, such as alfalfa, blue green algae, apricots, cantaloupe, carrots, dandelion, collard greens, garlic, parsley, pumpkin, yams, tomato, red pepper, and sweet potato. Legumes, grains and seeds also contain a significant portion of carotene. Vitamin A may be helpful therapeutically for diabetes, high cholesterol, gout, infections, conjunctivitis, and dry skin.

—**Vitamin B complex.** All of the B-vitamins are water-soluble and can be cultivated from bacteria, yeasts, molds, or fungi. There are eight B vitamins: B1 (thiamine), B2(riboflavin), B3(niacin), B5 (pantothenic acid), B6 (pyridoxine), B12 (cobalamin), folic acid, and biotin. The B vitamins are necessary for healthy nerves, thyroid function, heart, muscles, immune system, eyes, skin, feathers, liver, red blood cell formation, cell growth and reproduction, and to promote proper digestion. The B vitamins work as a team and are codependent for effectiveness. They provide the body with energy by assisting enzymes in the metabolism of carbohydrates, fats and proteins. Some factors which deplete the B vitamins from the body are stress, antibiotics or sulfa drugs, and excess sugar. A deficiency may cause dry skin and feathers, maldigestion, appetite loss, fatigue, constipation, cataracts (B2), weakness and depression. These vitamins may be easily obtained by feeding whole-grains, seeds, nuts, legumes, brewer's yeast, green vegetables, eggs, and yogurt, and intestinal bacteria produce the B vitamins as well. The B vitamins may be beneficially therapeutic for gout, blood sugar disorders, digestive disturbances, and stress.

—**Vitamin C** (ascorbic acid). This vitamin is a natural anti-inflammatory, antihistamine, antioxidant, and anti-stress nutrient. It assists in collagen production, iron absorption, red blood cell formation, proper function of the adrenal glands, burn and wound healing, and boosts immune system function. The absorption of iron and calcium are increased by adequate intake of vitamin C. Foods high in vitamin C work as antioxidants which help free the body of the daily toxins (unavoidable in some cases) which are in our air, water, some foods, radiation, toxic metals, stress, and other harmful environmental conditions (known as "free radicals") which cause damage to our birds' health. Since birds are known to manufacture vitamin C in sufficient amounts, many feel it is not necessary to supplement their diet. We have noticed at times of stress, and that includes at breeding times, our birds consume larger amounts of foods containing this vitamin, thus, we feel it to be especially useful at these times. Also, a bird may have a dysfunction of the enzyme which produces vitamin C, therefore individual requirements may vary. This vitamin is known to prevent *C. albicans*, viral and various bacterial infections. Some factors which deplete vitamin C from the body are stress, air pollution, cortisone, antihistamines, and tetracyclines. A deficiency may cause anemia, poor digestion, decrease resistance to infections, stress, bone and joint disorders, and dry skin and feathers. Vitamin C is found in citrus fruits, berries, green leafy vegetables, potatoes, tomatoes, peppers, garlic and most fresh uncooked fruits and vegetables. Vitamin C therapy may help with allergies, high cholesterol, sinusitis, diabetes, gout, heart disease, cataracts, gout, cancer prevention, and kidney disorders.

—**Bioflavonoids.** These nutrients are not synthesized by the body and must be obtained in the diet. There are many different bioflavonoids, including hesperidin, quercetin, rutin and they are sometimes referred to as vitamin P. Bioflavonoids possess anti-oxidant, anti-inflammatory and anti-allergenic properties. They often occur with vitamin C in fruits and vegetables as they work in conjunction with vitamin C to enhance its absorption. Bioflavonoids are found in the pulp and white rind just beneath the peel of citrus fruits, along with cherries, blackberries, blueberries, apricots, grapes, peppers, soybeans, garlic, and buckwheat. Bioflavonoids may be helpful for reducing pain, healing bruises, protecting the structure of the capillaries, and have been known to possess antibacterial properties, and aid in the prevention of cataracts and cancer.

—**Vitamin D.** This fat soluble vitamin can be synthesized by the body by exposing the skin to the ultraviolet rays of the sun or included in the diet by consuming foods or supplements which contain this vitamin. The interaction of the ultraviolet rays with a bird's preening oils, which contain 7-dehydocholesterol, aids in the conversion of vitamin D. Full spectrum lighting also provides exposure to ultraviolet rays. These lights are often used in bird rooms and aviaries as an artificial substitute for sunlight. Provitamins D are found in both plant and animal tissue.

Vitamin D is important for the absorption of calcium from the intestines, and in the breakdown and assimilation of phosphorus. It is also necessary for the normal depositing of these minerals into bones and for normal growth and development. Vitamin D in conjunction with calcium is valuable in maintaining a stable nervous system, normal heart action, thyroid function, normal blood-clotting, and proper egg-shell formation.

Excess vitamin D can be toxic, creating hypervitaminosis D, resulting in calcium reabsorption from bone and its redepositing in soft tissues, such as of the lungs or heart, and kidney damage. A deficiency may cause reduction in bone density, bone softening and fragility, rickets in growing youngsters, soft-shelled eggs, muscle spasms (tetany), diabetes, infection, conjunctivitis, stress, diarrhea, weight loss, skin and respiratory problems. Cortisone may deplete vitamin D from the body. Vitamin D is known to be an immunity enhancer and is best utilized when taken with vitamin A for a boost to the immune system. These two vitamins taken along with vitamin C act as a preventive measure against infection. Fish-liver oils are the best source of vitamins A and D, both which may possess anti-cancer properties.

—**Vitamin E.** A fat-soluble vitamin; E is used as a natural anti-allergic and antihistamine remedy. As an antioxidant, this vitamin protects the cells of the body against free radical damage from adverse environmental conditions. Vitamin E is known to speed healing (i.e., burns and wounds), strengthen the immune system, may prevent blood-clotting, helpful for the utilization of oxygen, and for the promotion of muscle and nerve maintenance. The most biologically active form is the natural d-alpha tocopherol. The synthetic form dl alpha has less nutritional value. Water-soluble E is available for those birds who have a liver or pancreas disorder or a fat malabsorption problem. Vitamin E is required in larger amounts if you live in an air-polluted area. A deficiency may cause intestinal disorders, dry skin and feathers, infertility, muscle weakness. Tocopherols occur in the highest concentrations in wheat germ oil, whole grains, raw seeds and nuts, green leafy vegetables, berries, tomatoes, eggs, and soybeans. Vitamin E has been recognized for its beneficial therapeutic effects against many health conditions such as cancer, heart and lung disease, liver disease, high cholesterol, diabetes, skin disorders, gout, cataracts, and infections.

—**Vitamin K.** This fat-soluble vitamin's main function is in the promotion of blood clotting. It is also useful for the normal functioning of the liver, and in the maintenance of strong bones. There are three main types: K1 (phylloquinone - from plants), K2 (menaquinone - synthesized from intestinal bacteria), and K3 (menadione) a water-soluble synthetic form that may be used for those who cannot utilize the natural form because of a liver or pancreas dysfunction or fat malabsorption problem. However, this form of vitamin K has been known to be toxic (M.C. Linder, 1991). For blood clotting purposes, any of the three vitamin K's are suitable. However, vitamin K1 appears to be superior in that it plays a significant role in bone health. A deficiency may occur from prolonged use of antibiotics or sulfa drugs, which destroy the "friendly" intestinal bacteria, air pollution, and X rays. A deficiency may cause impaired mineralization of bone and bone fragility. Acidophilus products may help to increase the beneficial intestinal flora and produce vitamin K2. Food sources of vitamin K1 are kelp, alfalfa, green leafy vegetables, eggs, and soybeans.

MINERALS: Minerals are involved in a variety of functions in the body and are classified as either major or minor (trace) based on intake level NOT on importance. They are necessary components of tissue, maintain fluid regulation, acid-alkaline balance, and are needed for construction of bone, blood formation, muscle contraction, nerve transmission, building protein, energy production, and many other processes. Balance and absorption of minerals are vital.

Plants incorporate minerals from the soil and form organic structures, which are easily digested. Fruits, green leafy vegetables, legumes, grains and seeds are often excellent sources of minerals if grown in mineral-rich soil. (Mineral deficient soil can cause the plant to take-up harmful substances such as aluminum.) We all depend on the quality of the soil with which our food is grown and only those vegetables grown in mineral-rich soils can have the capacity to nourish us and our birds properly.

—**Calcium.** The major function of calcium is to work in conjunction with magnesium and phosphorus for building and maintaining strong bones and in the metabolism of vitamin D. The ratio of calcium to phosphorus in bones is 2.5 to 1. Calcium also aids in enzyme function, fat metabolism, egg-shell formation, nerve transmission, hormonal secretion, blood clotting, muscle growth and contraction. It helps maintain a healthy heart and facilitates the passage of nutrients in and out of the cell walls. A high intake of calcium or vitamin D, or a parathyroid gland disorder is a potential source of *hypercalcemia* (an abnormally large amount of calcium in the blood). This may result in calcification of soft tissues, i.e., of the lungs or heart, and in bone disorders.

When purchasing a calcium supplement there are a few things to consider. Both dolomite and bone meal contain high concentrations of calcium and require sufficient production of hydrochloric acid in the stomach for its digestion and assimilation. They are *not* the easiest forms of calcium to absorb and may both be contaminated with lead residues. A liquid form consisting of calcium gluconate, calcium lactate, and calcium citrate is lower in strength, but readily absorbed.

Some factors which may deplete calcium in the body are lack of exercise, aging, stress, tetracyclines, a parathyroid gland disorder, insufficient vitamin D or an excess of refined sugar, protein, fat, phosphorus, or magnesium, and large amounts of foods containing oxalic acid. Calcium must always be balanced with phosphorus and magnesium with the addition of vitamin D3 for proper absorption. A low blood calcium level, known as *hypocalcemia,* could lead to impaired growth and the drawing of mineral from bone. As a result, a serious bone deformity called rickets could occur in youngsters. A reduction in bone density leading to weakness, bone softening and fragility could occur in adult birds. Other symptoms of hypocalcemia are muscle spasms, joint pain, seizures, heart disorders, elevated blood cholesterol, soft-shelled eggs, and nervousness. Food sources include yogurt, oats, buttermilk, legumes, nuts, some seeds (i.e., sunflower, sesame, pumpkin, almond), kelp, oranges, berries, parsley, and green leafy vegetables.

—**Phosphorus.** This mineral is primarily responsible for calcium absorption and utilization, RNA/DNA synthesis, energy production, nerve health, heart/muscle contraction, kidney function, enzyme activity, B vitamin utilization, and the utilization of fats, carbohydrates, and protein. Factors which inhibit phosphorus absorption are an excess of refined sugar, iron, and magnesium, and insufficient vitamin D and calcium. A deficiency may cause weight problems, joint stiffness, weakness, trembling, and appetite loss. Food sources include garlic, eggs, brewer's yeast, legumes, grains, seeds and nuts.

—**Magnesium.** This mineral aids mainly in bone growth, the function of nerves, blood sugar metabolism, muscles, the regulation of normal heartbeat, enzyme activation, acid-alkaline balance, protein synthesis, and energy reactions. It also assists with vitamin B, C and E utilization. Magnesium is located mostly in the bone with phosphorus and calcium with smaller amounts in cellular fluids and soft tissue. It helps with calcium, phosphorus, sodium, and potassium absorption and metabolism. Some factors which inhibit absorption of magnesium are stress, sugar, and tetracyclines. A deficiency may cause weakness, muscle tremors, weight loss, nervousness, feather loss. Food sources include whole grains, legumes, leafy greens, kelp, garlic, nuts, bananas, apricots, seeds. May be beneficial therapeutically for diabetes, high cholesterol, and heart disorders.

   —Potassium, Sodium, and Chlorine (Chloride). These minerals are electrolytes and they work together to maintain water balance, acid-base balance, and assists in muscle, nerve, heart, adrenal, liver and kidney function. Potassium is the major intracellular electrolyte. Sodium/chloride are found primarily in blood and the extracellular body fluids. Potassium and sodium regulate the transport of nutrients to the cells. Potassium assists in the metabolism of proteins and carbohydrates and activates certain enzymes. Sodium and chlorine aid digestion by stimulating the production of hydrochloric acid. Potassium may help treat diarrhea, blood sugar disorders, and heart disease. Excess sugar, stress, and cortisone may deplete potassium from the body. A deficiency may cause skin and feather problems, weakness, high cholesterol, nervousness, respiratory distress, appetite loss, weight loss, impaired digestion, sleepiness, decreased resistance to infection. Food sources of potassium include oranges, bananas, potatoes, seeds, legumes, yogurt, grains, chayote, yellow vegetables, parsley, yams, apricots, and dates. Food sources of sodium include celery, cheese, eggs, kelp. Food sources of chlorine include the same as sodium.

   —Sulfur. This mineral is part of the structure of certain amino acids, resists bacteria, and protects the protoplasm of the cells. Sulfur is prevalent in keratin which is found in the feathers, beaks, skin, and nails of birds. It is needed for the synthesis of collagen and stimulates the bile secretions of the liver. In addition, sulfur plays a part in tissue respiration, the process where oxygen and other substances function to build cells and to release energy. A deficiency may be caused by a low protein diet. This nutrient may be helpful for a variety of skin disorders, joint and intestinal problems. Food sources include eggs, garlic, kale, wheat germ, hot chili peppers, and legumes. Sulfur is also found in the B vitamins: thiamine and biotin.

Trace minerals:

—**Iron**. This mineral combines with protein and copper to assist with hemoglobin production and is required for stress and disease resistance. Tetracyclines may deplete iron from the body. A deficiency may cause anemia, fatigue, constipation, symptoms of stress, infection. Food sources include legumes, eggs, leafy veggies, kelp, seeds (sesame/sunflower/pumpkin), nuts (almonds), grains, and raisins.

—**Manganese.** This mineral aids in reproduction and growth, tissue respiration, bone development, a healthy immune system, vitamin B1 and vitamin E utilization, glucose regulation, fat and carbohydrate metabolism, energy production, and enzyme reactions. A deficiency may cause ataxia, elevated blood cholesterol, muscle weakness, blood sugar disorders, increased fat deposition. Food sources include eggs, grains, nuts, legumes, vegetables, blueberries, pineapple, and seeds.

—**Copper**. This mineral aids in the formation of hemoglobin, red blood cells, the production of collagen, protein metabolism, and is required for bone, blood vessel, nerve, joint, skin, immune system health. Zinc and vitamin C work in conjunction with copper and must be in proper balance for the formation of elastin. A deficiency may cause weakness, diarrhea, elevated blood cholesterol, immune system disorders, hypothyroidism, and skin and feather disorders. Food sources include legumes (soybeans), oats, potatoes, nuts, peas, and millet.

—**Iodine**. This mineral is necessary for normal cell metabolism, metabolism of excess fat, and thyroid function. A deficiency may cause goiter, hypothyroidism, obesity, dry, worn feathers, and fatigue. Food sources include kelp, sesame seeds, soybeans, and summer squash.

—**Cobalt.** This mineral is an important part of vitamin B12 and in the activation of enzymes. It is necessary for the proper function of red blood cells and in maintaining the health of the other body cells. A deficiency may cause anemia and nervous disorders. Food sources include spinach, beet greens, buckwheat, nuts, legumes, and figs.

—**Zinc**. This mineral assists with enzymatic reactions, carbohydrate digestion, facilitates the action of the B vitamins, circulation, liver function, immune system function, protein synthesis and cell growth, skin, bone, joint health, wound healing, and the growth of reproduction organs. Zinc also has antioxidant properties as does vitamin A, E, C and selenium and may help remove toxins from the body. Zinc increases the absorption of vitamin A which also strengthens the immune system. Therefore, a zinc deficiency could eventually lead to a vitamin A deficiency. However, if zinc were overdosed it can interfere with the proper function of the immune system and decrease vitamin A, copper, and iron stores. Toxicity can cause symptoms, such as loss of muscle coordination, fatigue, gastrointestinal disturbances, renal failure, and anemia. Large amounts of calcium may reduce the absorption of zinc. A high percentage of fiber in the diet will bind with zinc and remove it from the body before it has the chance to be absorbed. Cortisone may deplete zinc from the body. A deficiency may cause growth impairment, blood sugar disorders, fatigue, poor appetite, reproduction disorders, liver disease, infection, feather and skin problems. Food sources include peas, legumes, nuts, leafy vegetables, seeds (sesame/sunflower/pumpkin), egg yolks, and whole grains (sprouted).

—**Selenium.** This mineral is an important antioxidant, commonly combined with vitamin E. Selenium protects the immune system from damage by preventing the development of free radicals. Selenium and vitamin E work together to assist in the production of antibodies, amino acid metabolism, and assures adequate oxygen to the heart and a healthy liver. Selenium is also needed for proper pancreatic function and in the production of prostaglandins. A deficiency may cause reproduction disorders, blood sugar disorders, liver necrosis, cataracts, nerve disorders, repeated infections, and cancer. Food sources include eggs, sesame and sunflower seeds, whole grains, vegetables, and garlic.

Mineral supplementation. It is necessary to provide minerals in their proper amounts to prevent a negative effect on the body. Since we may not be able to administer the proper dosage of each individual mineral, it would be wise to consider purchasing a multi-mineral supplement. Four forms of minerals are currently available as supplements. Colloidal minerals are the largest. They are unable to penetrate the cell wall and can sometimes have detrimental effects on the body. Chelated are smaller and derived from plants which have already converted the mineral into a form the body can use. Ionic are smaller yet and have even more success at penetrating the cell wall. Crystalloid minerals are in the smallest form and can be absorbed into the cell wall most efficiently. It is necessary for minerals to penetrate the cell in order for them to efficiently perform their necessary functions. When shaken in water, these trace minerals create electrolytes to "charge" your bird's battery and keep his body electricity up to snuff!

An excellent way to give minerals to your bird is by adding them to their water. Water is a vital element to your bird's life. The body's water supply is responsible for and involved in nearly every body process including respiration, digestion, absorption, metabolism, excretion, and circulation. Water is also the primary transporter of nutrients throughout the body. Water helps maintain a proper body temperature and is necessary for carrying waste material out of the body. The functions water performs in the body will be compromised if minerals are not present in water (distillation and other processed water methods remove the minerals).

Unfortunately, the need to filter water has become a necessity because our public water supply contains many harmful pollutants (i.e., chemicals, metals, and microorganisms). There are many different types of water filter units on the market which are affordable. Choose one which has had a high rating for eliminating bacteria, parasites, chemical gases, lead, aluminum, chlorine, asbestos, nitrates, and pesticides. Selecting a unit that is equipped with a sub-micron ceramic filter will remove the above water contaminants and bacteria as well. After filtering your drinking water, the minerals should always be added back before giving it to your bird.

Water should also be supplied for bathing. A shower or bath is important to your bird's happiness and well-being. Filtered water should be used, especially if you are on a city water system that adds chlorine and fluoride to the water. Offer your bird a shower with a mister bottle or a compressed air sprayer, a minimum of three times a week in the winter months and daily, if you can, during the summer months. Occasionally, a bird may fear being misted if they are not accustomed to it and move quickly away from the watering device. With patience and time your bird will eventually realize that being misted is an enjoyable experience and look forward to the daily water-play with zest. The added moisture to your bird's feathers will promote preening activity for bright healthy feathers and also help to prevent dry skin.

Chapter 6
Health and Medicine.

"Most of the over-the-counter drugs and almost all prescribed drug treatments merely mask symptoms, control health problems, or in some way alter the way organs or systems such as the circulatory system work. Drugs almost never deal with the reasons why these problems exist while they frequently create new health problems as side effects of their activities."

--John R. Lee, M.D.

Many veterinarians still do not have an educational background in nutrition or natural healing protocols and must employ strong pharmaceutical drugs and/or surgery to treat their patients when an illness occurs. These doctors specialize in clinical medicine and surgery and are often experts in these methods; however, these methods are simply not always necessary and can often times do more harm than good with the side effects that they produce. When suppressive drugs are used for symptoms of illness, the condition may worsen to the point where a chronic or degenerative disease may result.

There are few cures in modern medicine, and for most conditions of illness. We are commonly just given a drug or two which can palliate the symptoms we are experiencing instead of being offered suggestions for better eating habits, balancing our biochemistry, and ways to strengthen our immune system to heal our body naturally. In certain cases, palliation may be a temporary or permanent answer if serious injury or pain occurs or if a bodily organ does not function properly. Palliation does not effect a cure, however, it can buy time in a life-threatening situation and does save lives. In extreme emergencies, fast-acting allopathic medicine/surgery may be relevant. This is when modern medicine is truly applicable.

With modern medical care, the root cause of illness is frequently ignored. If we are to strive for a true cure, then the emotional and mental symptoms are equally important to the physical symptoms that we experience. It is wise, therefore, to look at the whole picture of the malady to attempt to cure as often as possible, rather than to merely palliate the surface symptoms. If given the opportunity, nature is always our greatest healer.

Some of the illnesses and diseases our birds succumb to are remarkably similar to those that humans succumb to, such as cancer, diabetes, pancreatitis, hypothyroidism, kidney and liver disease, immune system disorders and the list goes on. Most health experts believe that modern medicine is not the best hope for most of our present health conditions, but that improvement to one's diet and environment are the number one factors which have the influence to bring us healthy living and increased longevity. While the foods we serve our birds will contribute largely to the quality of health they possess and help keep them disease-free, there are natural therapies which can aid in their recovery from illness, prevent disease, and reduce the stress they may experience at certain times in their lives. Regular exercise is also vital to your bird's good health and should be encouraged by purchasing the largest cage affordable and, if appropriate, allowing your bird supervised time outside of its cage. A cage or play area designed for interesting activities for your bird is the best way to prevent your bird from turning into a perch potato.

Drug-induced nutrient deficiency.

Many prescription drugs deplete nutrients. Drugs of any kind are always a trade-off. For every benefit, there are one or more drawbacks. Many drugs create vitamin and mineral deficiencies by blocking nutrient absorption, speeding excretion, or otherwise interfering with metabolism. We do not advocate the use of synthetic drugs, unless absolutely necessary. If there are natural, non-invasive, safe methods for overcoming illness then we utilize these first.

Natural methods for overcoming illness.

In our household, it is not the rule to run to a doctor for every complaint or ailment. We frequently are more likely to correct the imbalance or disharmony in the comfort of our own home. By asking ourselves many questions, thinking about what may have initiated our ailment, and then determining what we need for relief, we often find the cure and subsequently experience a quick recovery. For example, if one of us is feeling tired, stressed or a little "under the weather" we generally increase our vitamin C intake and increase our consumption of fruits and vegetables. Garlic may be used and vegetable juice for its detoxifying purposes. When our immune system has been pushed to the maximum and we feel we are not performing at our best we might use a product which includes astragalus, grapefruit extract, and echinacea to give us that extra boost. Probiotics and enzymes are also included in this regimen. Fresh air, sunshine, and relaxation also facilitate good health. Homeopathic medicines are consistently relied upon for illness or an injury for ourselves as well as for our pets and are an extremely effective healing modality. These are just a few examples of the remedies which can be very helpful.

I have translated many of the remedies which have been effective for us over to our animals and birds and have achieved remarkable results. Remember we are often our own and our pets best healers. Frequently we release this responsibility to an allopathic medical practitioner who is extremely limited in what he/she can offer us beyond lab work, (which may or may not be accurate) and routine drug prescriptions. With the guidance of a holistic veterinarian or other qualified individual there are many safe and effective natural methods to increase the vitality and improve the health of our birds

Homeopathic and Herbal First-Aid.

"The physician should speak of that which is invisible. What is visible should belong to his knowledge, and he should recognize the illness, just as everyone else, who is not a physician, can recognize them by their symptoms. But this is far from making him a physician; he becomes a physician only when he knows that which is unnamed, invisible, and immaterial, yet efficacious."
    -Paracelsus (1493-1541) Swiss physician and alchemist

Our bird's safety and wellness should always be a top priority. However, even the most scrupulous and watchful bird owners, who carefully look after their pet birds with every move they make, may not be able to prevent the occasional accident 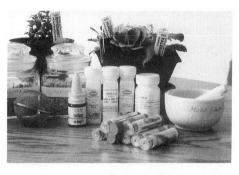 that can occur at a moment's notice. An accident might happen while our bird is in the "safety" of his or her own cage, at play on their play-gyms, or freely roaming about the room while we are enjoying some "quality time" with them. Accidents can happen whether or not our bird's wings are clipped, but most often seem to occur when they are not clipped properly. While every new bird owner should be sent home with a list of safe bird-keeping rules, many who have owned birds for years may need a little refresher course on accident prevention and the usefulness of a first-aid kit.

While a visit to our avian veterinarian may be the number one choice when our bird has been hurt or has become ill; there are many benefits to knowing the appropriate action to take in the case where your bird may have to wait to receive medical care and attention from a veterinarian. For instance, some bird owners may live several miles away from an avian veterinarian, the accident could happen in the middle of the night or on a holiday when a doctor is unavailable. It is a very secure feeling to have the products and materials handy when an emergency arises; having the knowledge and skill to use them properly is imperative. You may be able to begin the first-aid treatment prior to your veterinary appointment and it could buy you time until medical intervention is available. This knowledge just might help to save your bird's life!

Some of the best remedies I have utilized over the years for injuries, such as cuts, scrapes, wounds, bruises, trauma, fractures, stress, and the occasional illness have been homeopathic and herbal. I will list a few of the remedies that have been used successfully and hope that they may be useful to others in similar circumstances. This information is not meant to replace medical care by a knowledgeable avian veterinarian, but is for educational purposes only.

What is Homeopathy?
More and more people are becoming interested in natural health care. Herbal and homeopathic remedies can be very useful when an illness (both acute and chronic) or injury occurs. These remedies are favored for their safety and effectiveness and many of them have received scientific validation. Homeopathy is the oldest holistic system of medicine in the modern scientific era and has quite an extensive, interesting history.

In summary, this system of medicine was founded in the late 1700's by Samuel Hahneman, a German physician. However, it was Hippocrates who first discovered that certain herbs given in a low dose cured the same symptoms as they produced in a large dose. This was a time of much experimentation by Hahneman of this unique and profound theory and it was soon confirmed and instituted by many in the medical profession. The basic premise of homeopathy is that what in a large dose would cause disease symptoms in a healthy person would in a very small, infinitesimal dose, effect a cure in one who is ill. This highly systematic method includes the fundamental principles: *Law of Similars, use of a single remedy, and the minimum dose. The Law of Similars simply means "like cures like."* The word homeopathy was taken from Greek terminology; *homoios* meaning "similar" and *pathos* meaning "disease".

The classical form of homeopathy uses substances which are made from a single element; however, there are many combination (complex) remedies on the market. The substances used to make homeopathic remedies are generally either animal, mineral, or plant and are specially prepared by "potentization". Potentization consists of successive dilution and succussion (vigorous shaking of the mixture). Depending on the potency of a homeopathic preparation, you will see on the label, for instance, 6c, 30c, 200c. These are the most common strengths for first-aid care. The number indicates the number of times the remedy has been diluted and succussed. The c stands for centesimal potency (i.e., 1 part medicine to 99 parts diluent). Remember, while in a large, crude dose these substances would be harmful. On the contrary, in the low homeopathic dose are nontoxic.

When choosing a remedy the totality of the symptom picture is of primary importance. This means that not only are the physical symptoms acknowledged, but the mental and emotional ones too. Homeopathy takes many years of study to understand and use proficiently and as your interest grows in the learning of homeopathy there are many books to help aid your learning process.

Homeopathy for animals and birds has recently become quite popular with many veterinarians in the U.S. While in England, there are a number of veterinarians who regularly use homeopathic medicine for injury, illness and disease in animals and have done so for many years. There have also been a number of books published in England on veterinary homeopathy. Homeopathic remedies, are considered by many to be the ideal medicine because they help to stimulate the body's own natural defense mechanism, encourage maximum healing and well-being, and if used correctly do not simply palliate symptoms.

Many bird owners are interested in helping their pets to heal with a nutritional and natural approach, as they do for themselves.

Often times pet owners are the best healers because they know their pets so well. Understandably, however, beginners are often reluctant to try something new for their pet and need education in these areas to bring about a level of confidence before attempting to use an unfamiliar product or remedy. Learning about homeopathic first-aid is a great way to get started in understanding one of the most popular holistic healing arts today!

I hope the following remedies will be useful to you for a variety of problems should they be indicated. I have listed a few resources at the end of this book which are meant to help guide you in gaining more knowledge. You may also seek assistance from a veterinary homeopath experienced with birds for additional advice. Remember, these remedies may be used in conjunction with allopathic medicine should they be necessary. Please note that some remedies will be used topically (ointment), orally (globules, pillules, tablets) or both... depending on the injury.

—**Arnica.** (Mountain daisy) Anti-inflammatory, vulnerary. Helps with physical and emotional trauma and stress from injury. Good for sprains, fractures, and bruises. Reduces pain and swelling. *Arnica* ointment may be used externally if skin is not broken. Egg binding (vet care recommended). Useful before and after surgery. *Ruta* treatment may be indicated following *Arnica* for stiffness in wings and legs during healing. 6c or 30c as needed.

—**Euphrasia.** (Eyebright) an astringent. Very helpful for eye infections (conjunctivitis), irritation, or inflammation. Make an herbal infusion; use as an eyewash. Homeopathic remedy may also be offered orally, 30c.

—**Calendula.** (Marigold) antiseptic, analgesic, anti-inflammatory herb. Heals skin wounds, cuts, abrasions, and minor burns. Stops bleeding and promotes healthy tissue repair. Heals umbilicus (navel) in neonates. After proper cleansing, apply herbal ointment (may also include *Echinacea*, vitamin E, comfrey, red clover, burdock root, mugwort, etc.). Homeopathic remedy may also be offered orally, 30c.

—**Belladonna.** (Deadly nightshade) heatstroke, 30C. Misting your bird with cool water will also help to lower its body temperature.

—**Hypericum.** (St. John's Wort) antiseptic, analgesic, stops bleeding, healing agent. Helpful for injuries and nerve damage of the feet, toes, and claws. Used after amputation of a limb to promote healing. Relieves pain from injury. Useful for burn accidents following oral *Cantharis*. May be used in conjunction with *Calendula* ointment, such as Hypercal®, orally 30c.

—**Cantharis.** (Spanish-fly) used for burns. Apply cold water compress, then oral dose *Cantharis* 30c every hour as required. If distress accompanies burns *Arnica* or *Aconite* 30c may be indicated, followed by *Calendula* or *Hypericum* externally. Appropriate gauze dressing and bandaging should be applied. *Aloe vera* gel is also highly effective in soothing and healing burns.

—**Ruta Graveolens.** (Rue) for stiff or sprained limbs during recovery from injur, 6c.

—**Rhus Toxicodendron.** (Poison ivy) stiff, swollen, painful joints and limbs, 6c or 30c.

—**Aconite.** (Monkshood) indicated for injury and shock where there is fear. Useful after unexpected temperature extreme or exposure to cold wind. Also, used for respiratory distress.

—**Ledum.** (Marsh tea) used for skin injuries, puncture wounds from cat scratches and inflammation. 6c or 30c orally. Use *calendula/hypericum* (Hypercal®) ointment topically.

—**Ignatia.** (St. Ignatius' bean) indicated for sorrow or fear and loss of a mate or owner. For very stressed, nervous bird, 30c.

—**Symphytum.** (Comfrey) following *Arnica* for trauma. Heals and aids speedy recovery to fractured bones or wings. Useful in the stimulation of bone, connective tissue and cartilage repair. Use after bones/wings have been set. Calc Phos (Phosphate of lime) 6c or 30c, may be used to complete union of severe fracture. *Symphytum* is also helpful for eye injuries, 6c or 30c.

—**Manganum Aceticum.** (Manganese acetate) good for sore, swollen feet after limb injury, 30c.

—**Allium Cepa**. (Onion) may be indicated for your friends or relatives who may be allergic to your feathered friend's dander. Give them a dose of 30c to relieve symptoms such as sneezing and runny, burning eyes, better in open air.

NOTE: When using homeopathic pills, crush into fine powder. This powder may be mixed with a little distilled or filtered water before placing into beak by eyedropper or syringe. Offer remedy away from mealtime. Once a remedy has shown its effectiveness, you should discontinue its use.

There are many other homeopathic and herbal remedies available for those who prefer natural healing versus allopathic treatment. It is most important to determine what ailments require which type of treatment, or a combination of both. By using the appropriate alternative medicine, we find we are often able to avoid a stronger, more powerful allopathic medicine, thus eliminating the concerns we have of their direct negative effects on our birds' bodies. However, if allopathic medicines are needed in a life-threatening situation, then we should not hesitate to utilize them.

Additional supplies to have handy at all times.

Q-tips, cotton balls, gauze pads, tweezers, vetwrap bandaging tape, first-aid tape, scissors, hydrogen peroxide or betadine solution, toothpicks and popsicle sticks (splints), syringes/eyedroppers, needle-nosed pliers (for pulling broken blood feathers), heating lamp, cornstarch/flour (to stop bleeding), and an electrolyte solution.

Chapter 7
Stress Reduction Naturally.

Immune system and stress.

When we talk about stress we must also invariably talk about the immune system. Immune deficiencies are one of the problems commonly found with breeding and pet birds, and often stress plays a major role in this disorder. The immune system is essentially made up of white blood cells called B cells and T cells. B cells produce antibodies that aid in the attack of bacterial or viral infections. T cells are responsible for cellular immunity against a variety of illness and disease, such as fungi, parasites, and viruses. When incorporating the proper foods, vitamins, minerals and specific medicinal herbs we increase the activity and/or number of T and B cells which keep our bird's body healthy and strong. By implementing the suggestions in this book, along with providing a clean, comfortable environment, we greatly improve our birds constitution, help relieve stress and build better function of their immune system.

The anatomy of stress.

Problems related to stress or anxiety may manifest in only psychological and behavioral ways or in physical symptoms, such as self-mutilation of feathers or infection. Stress can cause many types of disease as there is a link between emotional and physical illness. The symptoms of this imbalance are usually emotional at first (agitation) then may become physical (feather-picking) and may eventually lead to illness (bacterial, viral, or organ damage). We and our birds are all carriers of yeast, bacteria and viruses, but they remain in small amounts and harmless under healthy conditions. However, at stressful times when the immune system is weakened, these opportunistic microorganisms may proliferate and our birds then become more vulnerable to the development of an infection. These microorganisms are the result of dis-ease, NOT the cause of it.

When our bird is experiencing stress either physically or emotionally, its metabolic response to this stress is to activate the sympathetic nervous system. This is a component of the autonomic nervous system which prepares the body for action during the fight or flight response. Some of the physiological changes which take place are increased sugar and fats into the bloodstream, the production of more adrenaline, cortisol, and glucagon into the blood, a decrease in the digestive function, increased blood pressure, heartbeat, breathing rate, muscle tension, and thus the creation of more energy.

In our bird's captive environment there is usually little physical outlet for them other than chewing (sometimes themselves), eating, playing with "toys", climbing, or sometimes flying about their cage. Consequently, the bird may react to stress by channeling the body's response to physical destruction, such as feather picking itself or a cage mate, which are often quite difficult to eradicate once it becomes a normal psychological response to stress. Stress may also manifest itself inward to one of the organ systems, such as the nervous system, circulatory, or digestive system. Stress increases the metabolism of proteins, fats, and carbohydrates. There is an increased excretion of amino acids, potassium, and phosphorus and a decreased storage of calcium. Vitamin C and other important nutrients are also excreted at a faster rate. During stress, nutrients are depleted from the body rapidly and the immune system becomes depressed. In essence, when our birds are under stress, the whole body is affected.

A proper diet is extremely important as disorders which can arise from stress are often the result of nutrient deficiencies; the body does not metabolize nutrients well at these times. Chronic stress can harm the nervous system, thereby causing digestive and intestinal upsets. Stress also leads to hormonal imbalances---adrenal, pituitary, thyroid, thymus and others that further interfere with immune function. Respiratory infections, allergies, eating disorders, diarrhea, skin and feather problems are a few of the outward symptoms of stress, therefore additional supplements are useful.

Etiology of stress.

It is very helpful to investigate and detect any subtle, or not so subtle disturbances/changes/threats in your bird's environment which may be causing stress. Is your bird experiencing any of the following psychological or biological problems or adverse environmental conditions?

After reading through the following list, think about how you can improve any of the things you feel may be negatively affecting your bird's life: a new pet, family member, or guest in the home; a new cage/cage mate; rearrangement of furniture, remodeling of your home, or new household items, (i.e., furniture, drapes/blinds, etc.); a nutritional deficiency/excess/imbalance; digestive stress; metabolic disorder; an infection; medication; nervous system disorder; genetic factors; metal toxicity; environmental toxins (pesticides, herbicides, fungicides and other air pollutants); food intolerances or allergies to specific ingredients, (i.e., chemical preservatives, sugar, artificial colorings/flavoring, etc.) [any of these substances may cause hyperactivity]; water contaminants; hygiene neglect (i.e., dirty cage, infrequent bathing opportunity); lack of exercise (a cage too small); sorrow from the loss of a loved one (owner/mate); social stress, (i.e., insecurity from frequently absent owner, inconsistent attention from owner).

Other causes of stress are: erratic feeding schedule; loneliness; fear; excess noise; over stimulating environment; insufficient rest; travel, cage relocation, move to a new home; seasonal changes, temperature extremes; breeding tension (i.e., the inability to satisfy breeding urges; the raising and caring for young, baby or egg removal); boredom; disturbance from rodents, insects, wild birds, or household pets. A traumatic event like being mishandled, abused by a former owner, or groomed incorrectly by an inexperienced person can also initiate stress. Any of these stress factors may be causing your bird's uneasiness. Determining the cause requires your ongoing observation and keen insight in order to adjust the situation to alleviate the stress-causing factor(s) as soon as possible. Knowing your bird's history, such as the diet and care it once received, is vital for properly understanding the stress symptoms it may be experiencing today.

A few tips.

Remember some stress-related cases are easier than others to correct. Begin with the generalities of the individual bird's situation and then narrow them down to specifics. For instance, take note of when (time of day) and where (location) is your bird noticeably experiencing stress symptoms, (i.e., feather chewing/picking)? Is the diet you are feeding providing optimum health for your bird or is it only maintaining its health? Does the diet contain additives which may be causing exciting effects? Is your bird uncomfortable with its environment in any way (i.e., location of cage, perches, food bowls)? Is there an object or toy within the cage that frightens your bird or is there something outside its cage that may be causing its discontentment? These are just of few of the questions that you can ask yourself. Remember the main focus should be on the underlying cause of stress, instead of the stress symptoms.

Our birds seem to be more prone to stress by nature with their sensitive, intelligent personalities, and require we take their emotional health, as well as their physical health into consideration. In this way, we are truly using a holistic approach for their health needs and are far more likely to succeed in providing them with a stress-free life. I hope the following supplements will be useful for stress reduction for your pet or breeder bird.

Herbal supplements.

Nature has provided us with many plants which can benefit the nervous system, boost immunity, and reduce stress. There are herbs which can be successfully used for our birds to prevent the need for potentially toxic synthetic psychotropic drugs and other invasive means. Whether it be the nervous system or the immune system that becomes compromised, natural medicine has much to offer to aid in the recovery from stress. For chronic feather plucking caused by stress the typical allopathic treatment is one which is suppressive, not curative. I would always rather see a natural remedy used for behavior modification, than a synthetic drug which is potentially damaging to the health of any pet. Herbs can be one way to safely ameliorate stress, but will also be palliative and rarely remove it. They may exert a calming and restful effect when dealing with stressful situations, but will often require you also seek help from various caring professionals (i.e., veterinarian, nutritionist, or behaviorist) who specialize in birds, to help discover the root cause of the stress your bird is experiencing.

If you desire holistic veterinary care, information on any medicine prescribed by your allopathic vet, must be released to your holistic veterinarian who will take this into consideration prior to the selection of a natural therapy. The detoxification of an allopathic drug is often begun immediately through diet and vitamin therapy. If your bird is being treated for a chronic disease, your holistic veterinarian may prescribe a remedy or treatment, which will work positively in conjunction with this medicine. If possible, they will slowly wean your bird from the allopathic medicine to the use of a natural remedy or therapy.

The following herbs are used to calm our birds and provide them some relief during times of stress and are easily incorporated into their diet. Best known for their calmative properties, and also known as nervines are chamomile, passion flower, oat straw, skullcap, valerian, kava kava, lemon Balm, St. John's wort, and Siberian ginseng. They are some of the more common herbs used for managing stress. Oat straw, lemon balm, kava kava and St. John's wort are noted for their mild anti-depressive abilities. Certain herbs, such as ginseng are known as adaptogens which help us cope with stress and a changing environment in a positive way. Herbs which can strengthen and balance the functioning of the nervous system, hormonal system and consequently affect the immune system are also known as adaptogens. An adaptogen enhances adrenal gland function, possibly pituitary gland function, relaxes or equalizes the nervous system, and improves the body's reactions against a variety of stressors whether they be metabolic, physical or psychological in nature.

We purchase the above listed herbs in capsule form or liquid extract. These products have been standardized or quality controlled for optimum results. They may also be purchased fresh-dried in the bulk herb section of a natural food store or home-grown. Herbal supplements are generally available in a combination of two or more herbs or sometimes as a single herb remedy. We have found valerian/passionflower to be the most helpful for advanced stress-related feather-picking. Be sure treatment is given no longer than 2 weeks at a time. The other calmative herbs listed have been helpful for mildly stressed non-feather-picking birds.

The echinacea herb is highly regarded for its use as a natural antibiotic and immunity enhancer. By far the quickest and simplest way to provide an herb to your bird's diet is in capsule form. We use a combination herbal preparation consisting of: echinacea, astragalus, and grapefruit extract.

An herbal extract, which tends to be more potent then capsule powder, is offered over fresh food, mixed in formula, mixed in drinking water, or diluted with filtered water or organic apple juice and offered by syringe. We use an alcohol-free extract of echinacea, goldenseal, and vitamin C.

Herbs in the fresh-dried form (stems/leaves/flowers) can be made into liquid by infusion - (place 1-2 tsp. of dried herbs into infusion ball (stainless steel or porcelain) then place in 1 cup of boiling water, steep for 10-15 min.) or by decoction - (seeds/root/bark should be crushed or cut and boiled for 20 min).

Serve liquid warm. When preparing herbs in this way we offer by syringe, add to the handfeeding formula, or to the water source. Always begin by offering herbs in minute amounts and increase gradually. When illness is caught in the early stages and the proper products are given immediately, we can often expect a quick recovery.

When using herbs, it is wise to determine whether the compound is to be used therapeutically or tonically. If an herb is to be used therapeutically (for acute illness/infection/stress) it is best to use it for a short period of time (1 to 2 weeks) or five days on, five days off, etc. while reevaluating your bird's overall health. While used as a tonic (for chronic illness/infection/stress) it is best to use for a longer period of time for its mild effects and ongoing benefits. Dosages will vary from bird to bird and may be adjusted over time.

Another method, used for adult birds is the "herbal mist" --a very simple preparation of an herbal infusion or decoction with the herb(s) of choice. Pour the liquid into a clean mister bottle and shower each bird thoroughly. We use 4 cups of water to 3 tsp. of dried herb. Offered warm it acts as a nebulizer/drink, soothing the mucous membranes, which provides improved respiratory function, while being a refreshing experience for your birds. Your birds will also consume some of the herb while preening themselves. The herbal infusion/decoction can be kept fresh in the refrigerator for 2-3 days and be offered chilled in the warmer months. We sometimes offer our birds just a sprig or two of a particular herb fresh from our garden, but just like anything new, your birds may be skeptical. Some herbs are sweet, others bitter, your birds will certainly let you know which ones they like or don't like! Disguising the herb(s) may be necessary in cases where they continuously refuse them. This is accomplished by mixing or mashing thoroughly in a fresh food meal. The fresh herbs our parrots receive are in our "mash" diet, or sprinkled on top, and so are readily consumed. Herbs also contain varying amounts of vitamins and minerals and provide nutritional support so vital in times of stress.

An effective treatment for stress is to administer flower remedies that work directly on the emotions. Five flower essence combinations contain Cherry Plum, Clematis, Impatiens, Rock Rose, and Star of Bethlehem. For example, before and after a veterinary visit, place two drops of a five flower essence in 1 oz. of distilled or filtered water, shake well, offer 1-2 drops on tongue.

Nutritional supplements.

The adrenal glands are the most affected by stress and require that we offer higher levels of the following anti-stress foods/supplements to support their function. The vitamins and minerals which are effective in reducing stress in your bird's life are the B complex vitamins (particularly B5, the anti-stress vitamin and B6). Nutritional yeast, seeds, legumes, and grains are excellent B vitamin sources. Vitamin C including bioflavonoids (citrus fruits, berries, melons, kale, collards, parsley, potatoes, tomatoes, sweet potatoes, peas) vitamin E (nuts, grains, seeds, wheat germ oil,) and essential fatty acids (seeds, nuts, grains, flax seed oil, and evening primrose oil) are beneficial for strengthening immunity which is lowered at stressful times. Let's not forget vitamin A (in many veggies and fruits) for its ability to strengthen the cell walls, protect the mucous membranes and prevent allergies, thus helping your bird's body resist infection at times of stress when resistance is lowered. This vitamin is particularly helpful to those birds who are prone to respiratory problems.

The amino acid useful during intense stress is tyrosine, while the amino acid tryptophan is known for its calming effect. Be sure quality protein foods such as seeds/nuts, grains/legumes/greens combined) are a part of the diet. Foods, such as vegetables, legumes and grains are rich in potassium, calcium, magnesium, and zinc. Maintaining proper levels of these minerals are very important during stressful times. We also use an electrolyte solution which contains several valuable minerals. This can be added 50/50 to water. Stress uses up the minerals in your bird's body and replenishing them is essential. We use a calcium magnesium liquid, with natural vitamin D3 for its calming effect on the nervous system, particularly during stress. Air cleaners, such as the HEPA (High Efficiency Particulate Arresting) or the ozone air purifiers have also been found to be helpful in stress elimination.

Recognizing or even anticipating stressful situations helps to ease the times which are fraught with change, anxiety, fear, or even depression. If a period of stress is unquestionably about to occur, you can plan ahead by having proper supplements on hand. By providing additional vitamins, minerals, amino acids, soothing herbs, the proper foods and positive life-style changes, we go a long way in making the transitions in our bird's life more tolerable and help them to handle stress more effectively. Then all we need to add in love...

Chapter 8
Nutritional Therapy for Gout.

There are two forms of gout: articular gout, where urate deposits affect the hock and foot joints and visceral gout where urate deposits are found most frequently on internal organs, such as the liver, kidney, pericardium, heart, and air sacs. Symptoms may include weight loss, fecal inconsistency, and fatigue. Sometimes both forms are seen together in a patient. Gout, a form of arthritis, is classified as a metabolic disorder and is associated with high blood levels of uric acid which is the end product of purine (organic compounds found in certain foods) and protein metabolism. In articular gout, uric acid is deposited in the form of monosodium urate crystals in the tissue around the joints. This can cause inflammation of the joint, resulting in irritation, stiffness, severe pain, and may lead to joint deformity. A whitish stain may be seen on the feet or whitish-yellow subcutaneous nodules called tophi. While there is no known "cure" it may be controlled by diet and the decrease of purines, proteins, and sugars.

Gout may be caused by an amino acid imbalance causing too much uric acid to be produced. The body does not have the ability to breakdown proteins efficiently (possible liver dysfunction), kidney disorder, stress, sugars, obesity, improper diet, infection, certain drugs, such as antibiotics, the over-activity of the enzyme xanthine oxidase, or can often times be hereditary. In some cases, hypothyroidism patients have a high uric acid level with or without gout.

Dietary recommendations would consist of offering a variety of fruits and vegetables to help eliminate the uric acid. Also seeds, grains, nuts, and sprouts are excellent foods to provide your bird because they contain quality protein without the uric acid build-up. Herbs, such as Burdock, Devil's Claw, and Saffron neutralize uric acid. Dandelion is especially good for detoxifying the liver and filtering uric acid from the kidneys. Garlic may help the kidneys to eliminate uric acid. We use aged garlic extract, an odorless capsule powder or liquid. Charcoal capsule powder mixed into fresh food may be helpful in reducing uric acid levels. Vitamin C with bioflavonoids helps to lower serum uric acid levels. Water intake is very important for flushing out the uric acid excess. Vitamin E improves circulation and helps along with vitamin A to prevent toxin accumulation in the joints. An essential fatty acid supplement such as flax seed oil helps repair and heal tissues; mix one tbs. per lb. of seed. Kelp granules and alfalfa powder are rich in minerals and also promote healing. B complex helps with stress, circulation, and protein metabolism.

➡Foods which should be fed on a limited basis are legumes, meats, fish, asparagus, poultry, eggs, oatmeal, cooked spinach, cauliflower, peas, white flour, sugar products, and any processed feed high in protein as these foods contribute to uric acid formation.
➡Processed foods which contain a high level of sucrose, corn syrup, molasses, or high-fructose corn syrup should be avoided because they increase the production of uric acid, weaken the immune system, and adversely affect pancreatic function. If a bird has a predisposition to gout then fruit sugar should also be limited in the diet.

The common cherry, Prunus avium, containing keracyanin, has helped maintain normal uric acid levels in gout patients before the introduction of synthetic therapy. Other berries, such as strawberries and blueberries may be helpful as well. A **cherry fruit extract** supplement may be beneficial.

Conventional medical treatment.

Most often an anti-inflammatory drug such as cortisone is prescribed to reduce the swelling, but this drug may adversely affect the adrenal glands. However, there are drugs which can lower the urate levels by inhibiting the formation of uric acid. Allopurinol is sometimes used to control gout by impeding uric acid synthesis, but may cause serious side effects such as liver disease, eye damage, skin rash, diarrhea, sleepiness, or even worsen the gout condition. Also, this drug is contraindicated if kidney problems exist. (Conversely, if gout is not treated it can lead to kidney disease.) This drug is normally used in advanced cases. The medical treatment will depend on how severe the condition is and how well the patient is responding to the dietary changes.

Homeopathic remedies.

Those which may help reduce pain are: Rhus Tox 30c, Ledum pal 30c, Bryonia alba. 30c.

Chapter 9
Natural Prevention and Treatments for Candida.

What follows is our experience on how certain natural remedies can control and prevent *Candida albicans* (yeast) in birds and particularly in the neonate and young birds which have not yet weaned.

Yeast is a unicellular (single-celled) microorganism, a member of a sub group of the family of plants, known as fungi or mold, and reproduces by budding. It survives in most organic sources or anything alive and its reproduction is rapid. As humans, we have yeast in our bodies at all times, and in small amounts it is quite normal. It is when there is an imbalance of the intestinal ecology, by the use of antibiotics, for example, which destroys the "friendly" bacteria in the small intestine, that *C. albicans* can go from a simple form to a mycelial (rootlet) form causing negative symptoms (allergic and toxic reactions) and then treatment becomes necessary.

Some individuals may be more prone to a yeast infection due to handfeeding implements and the dark, warm, humid environment, they must be placed in as babies. Particularly in young birds and in certain avian species (i.e., lories and lorikeets), which have a high sugar diet, we commonly find problems with yeast. Foods containing refined carbohydrates cause yeast cells to increase. Those products containing a high percentage of sucrose or corn syrup are not healthful and contribute to a variety of illness. An alternative to "white sugars" are whole grain sweeteners (e.g., barley malt and brown rice sugars) or organically grown Sucanat.

C. albicans is classified as an "opportunistic" infection, meaning it can only flourish in an immune depleted environment. The most common areas for *C. albicans* to spread in a bird are in the mouth, tongue, pharynx, larynx, esophagus, and throughout the intestinal tract. Visually, it appears as a white, cheesy exudate and often has a foul odor. The crop may become distended with a fluid and mucous content, giving a balloon-like appearance. In many cases, bacterial symptoms will be observed such as a fluid discharge from the nasal passages and eye ducts. Further complications can exist such as crop stasis, vomiting, swallowing problems and/or beak deformities.

Diagnosis.

Choanal and cloacal cultures are done to determine whether yeast or other pathogens are present. A blood test which shows an abnormally high white blood cell count indicates an infection. Another diagnostic tool is a blood test which can detect *C. albicans* by checking for precipitins (antibodies) by double immunodiffusion. When these precipitins are detected, it is clearly evident that this organism is present and creating an active infection. If parasites are present this may inhibit the recovery of a yeast infection, therefore a parasite test is recommended as well.

C. albicans is one of the most dealt with and common ailments in birds and we feel strongly that we can ameliorate this illness without treatment with antifungals such as Nystatin, Nizoral, etc. These drugs (and others) can only over time become damaging to the birds being treated, while the yeast your birds are carrying may also build a resistance to these drugs as the organisms mutate into another species of yeast. It has been reported that *C. albicans* is now becoming resistant to the common antifungals, such as Nystatin. Furthermore, Nystatin can only kill the yeast for which it comes in direct contact with, so may be useless in cases where the yeast is dispersed throughout the entire intestinal tract.

This leads to much frustration for those bird owners and breeders whose bird(s) seem to have a chronic illness. These birds are repeatedly placed on an antifungal for yeast, and if bacteria is present an antibacterial medicine, while their owners spend considerable amounts of money on tests of every kind possible in the search for an answer. A weak immune system is the underlying problem, which needs to be dealt with. We believe trying the alternative of natural therapy may make some meaningful difference in our aviaries. In general, a good diet consisting of fresh, clean, preferably certified organic foods. Fresh water (preferably filtered of impurities) along with a stress-free, clean environment will also reduce the chance for certain predisposing factors to set in and cause a rise in susceptibility in your bird's health.

In our experience, these drugs have not made an improvement, while a combination of the following products have completely cured *C. albicans* for our birds. Our goal is to try to hinder the process with which a bird can succumb to a chronic yeast problem; whereby, supplements to the diet may decrease the amount of these microorganisms in the bird's body.

Natural treatments.

We have had success in eliminating yeast infections with the use of Kaprycidin-A (coconut extract) or sometimes known as caprylic acid; a saturated fatty acid. Caprylic acid duplicates the same fatty acids produced by normal intestinal flora. It can destroy *C. albicans*, and as a result increases efficiency of the immune system. Effectiveness is equal or better to that of Nystatin, but it is a non-prescription medicine. If used in a time-release form, it is not absorbed from the small intestines, but passes through the intestinal tract, killing yeast with no side effects; however, it does have a slightly unpleasant odor. For adults, sprinkle on fresh food; for babies, mix sparingly in the handfeeding formula, increase gradually as baby grows. We've noticed immediate improvement (within 24 hours) when caught in the early stages.

I also recommend a high quality probiotic, such as *Lactobacillus acidophilus* or *Bifidobacterium bifidum*. For those who raise birds, these supplements are indispensable. Probiotics are particularly helpful for newly hatched chicks which are being hand reared from day one. This bacteria supplies them with the healthy intestinal flora and produces enzymes, which would normally be received by parent-fed chicks. These cultured products not only aid in digestion, but prevent many disorders, such as *C. albicans*, bacterial infections, and crop stasis, while also improving growth rates, because its increase in protein and calcium (and also vitamins B and K), created by the nature of culturing, is in a more bioavailable form.

Cultured products contain lactic bacteria, a single cell organism which occurs singly, in pairs, or in short chains and transforms sugar into lactic acid. Lactic acid can hinder the growth of *C. albicans*. Many pathogens cannot live in an acid medium, such as lactic acid. It helps to evacuate them by giving them less room to grow and competing with them for attachment sites. Lactic acid, acetic acid, formic acid, benzoic acid, and hydrogen peroxide are found in cultured products and they inhibit the function of the harmful microorganisms. The beneficial or "friendly" intestinal bacteria actually use the yeast cells as food. In addition, they help to assimilate food and its nutritional value more readily. It is known that birds do not possess the enzyme lactase and so can not break down and digest lactose products. The most important benefit of milk products transformed by *Lactobacilli* are that they are more easily digestible by the creation of the enzyme lactase. There are, however, milk-free *acidophilus* products available using a vegetable growing medium, but these apparently contain very little to none of the antibiotic benefits, as milk is a more nutritionally balanced medium. Yogurt is known to be the most effective in producing lactic acid.

Garlic, an historically known herb and a member of the lily family, has been used all over the world for centuries, but in more recent times is used as a nutritional supplement to achieve optimum health. Buying or growing it fresh can be used in only modest amounts due to its potent composition. The aged garlic extract which can be purchased in capsule powder or liquid is convenient to use. Garlic has the positive affect of cleansing the body systematically by its detoxifying ability. It is used as an anti-microbial agent to pathogenic bacteria, viruses, and yeast. It has also been used to treat wounds and to stimulate the immune system. It assists in improving circulation, lowers cholesterol levels, aids in digestion, and strengthens blood vessels. Its properties may also protect against liver disease, cancer, asthma, sinusitis (nasal congestion), gout, parasitic diarrhea (intestinal worms), *Proteus*, *Klebsiella*, *Pseudomonas*, *Aspergillus* and other fungi.

Once again, one of the biggest enemies to the "friendly" bacteria is the use of antibiotics. The use of broad spectrum antibiotics and steroids are problematic in that they can cause an increase in yeast, and the immune system becomes depressed. Many times synthetic drugs are too readily administered, even for minor conditions. There are many natural alternatives to these harsher drugs and these can often be just as effective, if not more so. As always, getting to the root cause and making the dietary and environmental changes necessary will ultimately cure disease and prevent its future recurrence.

While *acidophil* bacteria can be beneficial in treating enteritis and similar inflammations of the intestines, we have found the use of *Bifidobacteria* to be helpful for *E. coli*, which is commonly found in excess in young birds. These birds are often treated allopathically with Neomycin and other similar drugs. Certain strains of *E. coli* may build a resistance to these drugs, and as a result, these drugs will no longer be effective in eliminating this bacteria. Often the best cure is to strengthen the immune system by feeding a quality fresh food diet and offering natural supplements which also aid the immune system in a positive way.

Chapter 10
Avian Digestion and Natural Remedies for Crop Stasis.

The foods we feed our birds must be broken down either mechanically or chemically by their body into simpler forms so that they can be absorbed through the intestinal walls and transported by the blood to the cells. It is at this time that they provide our birds' production of energy and daily stamina. The avian digestive tract includes the proventriculus, gizzard, and the intestines (lower alimentary tract). The crop (upper alimentary tract), located in the lower neck, is an expandable organ; which provides a storage site for food waiting to be digested and utilized.

Essentially, a bird's undigested food passes through two chambers before reaching the intestines. The first creates the gastric juices, while the second performs the grinding process. The pancreas and the liver also aid in the digestion process. The pancreas secretes digestive enzymes for the digestion of starches, fats, and proteins. The liver secretes bile for the emulsification of fats in digestion and has many other functions related to the metabolism of nutrients.

The enzyme digestion of food is completed in the small intestine and the process ends with the products of digestion being absorbed through the intestinal wall and into the bloodstream. We have now reached the final stage of the digestive processes with the metabolism of the nutrients which underwent the chemical changes required for a healthy, growing bird. Some of these elements become stored in the body, while the rest are eliminated in fecal matter, through the large intestine. The fecal matter is an important symbol of health, by its texture and frequency, and sometimes color, though these can often times reflect the foods eaten. Signs of indigestion or disease can be recognized by a drastic change in the composition of the feces even though the same foods are consumed consistently (daily).

I receive many calls from fellow breeders and pet owners who are handfeeding and caring for a baby bird who has developed sour crop (crop stasis), or just a slow to empty crop; regurgitation of food or fluid may also occur. In the case of early discovery of a digestive disorder or a slow moving crop, first try to eliminate the possible causes. Was the formula too thick, not warm enough, was the baby fed too much sugar, protein, or fat, fed spoiled (check expiration dates) or poorly mixed formula? Is the brooder placed at the proper temperature and humidity?

These are the easier items to correct, but can sometimes be difficult to determine if you're a first time handfeeder. In the meantime, (depending on severity and other external symptoms) the following remedy may be helpful. The product of choice, in my opinion, is a quality probiotic (beneficial bacteria). These products aid in digestion, and bring about very quick results in most cases. The two products we use are a combination of *Lactobacilli acidophilus* and *Bifidobacterium bifidus*. Guidelines for dosage are 10g - 30g 1/8 tsp., 30g - 250g 1/4 tsp., 250g - 450g 1/2 tsp. First heat a little water to proper temperature, then add a small amount of the probiotics. Mix thoroughly, and feed small amounts, several times throughout the day as needed. After each serving gently massage the crop thoroughly; digestive normalcy should occur gradually. No food should be given for 24 hours unless all digestion has taken place. After approximately the 24 hour period, reevaluation of the bird's condition should be noted. If no signs of improvement are noticed, then a call to your avian veterinarian is in order. He/she may want to remove the crop contents which may possibly be bacteria infected. A Gram's stain and culture of your bird's choana and cloaca can determine if an infection is present. If a bacterial or fungal infection is diagnosed, it can be treated with a number of natural antibiotics and will generate no harmful side effects if used properly.

Probiotics inhibit the growth of many pathogens, including the common yeast infection, by producing lactic acid in the intestines; thereby improving intestinal health and promoting effective digestion. Lactic acid also helps with the absorption of calcium and other important minerals. This bacteria will additionally supply your bird with the good intestinal flora and produces enzymes, which would normally be received by parent-fed chicks. An enzyme supplement added to the handfeeding formula will aid digestion as well.

We don't recommend allopathic drugs, such as synthetic antibiotics or antifungals, unless they are absolutely necessary as they cause a decrease in the intestinal "friendly bacteria" resulting in a depleted immune system. Recurrence of a bacterial infection is possible as these bacteria are becoming resistant to antibacterial drugs. Once the "good" organisms are wiped out, it creates the perfect breeding ground for *Candida albicans*, for example. Last, but certainly not least, antibiotics contribute to diarrhea and nutrient loss.

Chapter 11
Herbal Medicine.

Before the advent of modern medicine many people knew about the beneficial components of herbs. Through trial and error it was discovered how certain herbs could achieve great success in relieving symptoms of illness. Many herbs contain powerful constituents that if 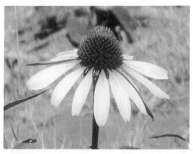 used correctly, can help with the healing process of disease and illness. Most herbalists agree that herbal medicine is just as effective as conventional medicine if used appropriately, but without the negative side effects. It is important to remember that not all plants possess healing properties and that there are as many poisonous plants as there are beneficial ones. Medicinal plants contain varying degrees of chemicals and have a direct impact on physiological activity. Taken internally, they activate overall body metabolism by providing a healing stimulus. Herbs also contain vitamins and minerals which are valuable to strengthen the constitution of the body at times of illness and stress. Herbs are generally used on a short-term basis (with the exception of certain herbs, such as garlic), and only as long as symptoms persist for a specific health problem. Sometimes herbal treatments are used for a longer period of time for chronic emotional or physical problems. We recommend you consult with a natural health care practitioner (avian specific), before the use of herbal medicine for your birds.

In our home, we are in favor of a holistic approach to healing. We have experienced a great deal of success with a variety of herbs for injury, illness and infection. Herbs can be purchased in many forms (i.e., liquid extracts, capsule powder, dried roots, leaves, or flowers and can be made into an infusion or decoction, eyewash/compress, ointment/salve). Administration of herbs can be achieved by sprinkling over fresh foods for self-feeding birds, offered by syringe for the care of an ill bird, or added to the handfeeding formula for a baby bird. Here, I will highlight for you a few of the herbs I use and their benefits.

—**Echinacea.** A bright and beautiful, purple daisy-like flower. It is one of the most commonly used herbs for strengthening the immune system and fighting infection. Echinacea is a native American herb that grows mainly in the plains of North America. The chemical constituents in Echinacea have anti-inflammatory abilities and destroy bacteria, viruses and other pathogens. Highly regarded for its antibiotic and immune enhancing activity, it has been indicated as a helpful remedy for respiratory distress as an anti-allergy treatment. The herb has been used in conjunction with immunosuppressing drugs and antibiotic therapy as a natural defense remedy. It also possesses the ability to prevent tumor growth. Echinacea is often used in combination with other herbs, such as goldenseal for viral, bacterial, and fungal infections. As an ointment or salve, it also helps to heal external wounds and may be used in a complex herbal formula.

—**Goldenseal.** A small native American perennial herb native to the North American woodlands, meadows, and mountain forests. This herb is used frequently for eye infections/irritation, digestive relief, appetite stimulation, liver disorders, diabetes, allergies/nasal congestion (sinusitis), and is used in cancer treatment against tumor growth. It is also used as a salve for its antiseptic qualities. Goldenseal possesses anti-microbial activity against *Salmonella*, *Chlamydia*, and has infection-fighting properties against yeast (*Candida*), bacteria, viruses, and protozoa, such a *Giardia*. It has also been found to act as a natural antihistamine. For serious ailments and emergency situations Echinacea and Goldenseal can be used in conjunction with other treatments.

—**Astragalus.** A Chinese herb that has been used for 2,000 years in China. Astragalus is used as an adaptogen and helps stimulate the immune system. It is often used before, during, and after times of stress and changes in one's lifestyle. This herb has been used in conjunction with immunosuppressing drugs as a defense remedy by increasing the number and activity of phagocytes in the blood and heightens the transformation of the lymphocytes into T-cells. The constituents of astragalus increase the activity of antibodies and are also effective in increasing cytokine activity, which inhibits viral reproduction. Astragalus helps the liver metabolize toxins, aids digestion, may improve lung damage and inhibit tumor growth.

—**Calendula.** An antiseptic, analgesic, and anti-inflammatory herb. Heals skin wounds, cuts, abrasions and minor burns. Stops bleeding and promotes healthy tissue repair.

—**Passionflower.** A calmative herb used in conjunction with other calming herbs, such as Valerian.

—**Valerian.** A nervous system relaxant. May relieve anxiety and stress-related disorders. The chemical ingredients in valerian are mild and much safer than conventional tranquilizing drugs.

—**Eyebright.** An astringent. Very helpful for eye infections (conjunctivitis), irritation, or inflammation. Used as an eyewash.

—**Garlic.** This herb is helpful as a digestive aid, may relieve respiratory distress, prevent and aid diarrhea, and is known to stimulate the immune system. Garlic has antibacterial, antifungal, antiviral, and antiparasitic properties. Aged Garlic Extract has been shown to have successful medicinal uses and is easy to administer if purchased in a liquid form.

—**Comfrey.** Valued as a demulcent herb it is rich in complex mucilage materials, which can soothe inflamed mucous membranes, and may improve respiratory distress. Aids digestive irritation and also aids speedy recovery to fractured bones when used *after* the bones have set by stimulating bone, connective tissue and cartilage repair. The herb is a helpful skin healing agent for wounds and burns. It is not advised for internal use for those with liver disease.

—**Pau d'arco.** This herb may ameliorate yeast, bacteria, allergies, diabetes, cancer, and liver disease in conjunction with other natural treatments.

—**Peppermint.** Used as a digestive aid, relaxant, may increase appetite, and aid diarrhea/intestinal disorders.

—**Thyme.** Helpful for allergies and nasal congestion (sinusitis). May help lower cholesterol.

Epilog.

Many birds suffer needlessly from improper nutrition, and a bird's diet is often what makes the difference between a healthy vibrant bird and one who is listless and unhealthy. Simply stated: It is my belief that improper foods create disease and that proper foods cure disease. We can solve many of our birds' health problems if we provide them with natural whole foods, a favorable environment, and the appropriate natural healing therapies.

Many aviculturists are recognizing the limitations of the commercial avian diets and the modern medical approach and are turning to natural methods for prevention and cure of disease. A natural diet and natural therapies stimulate and support the body's own inherent healing processes, which in turn leads to the ultimate goal we all wish to achieve... optimum health for our birds!

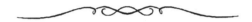

Resource Directory.

For a current list of holistic veterinarians, contact: **American Holistic Veterinary Medical Association**, 2214 Old Emmorton Rd. Bel Air, Maryland 21015 (410) 569-0795.

Product Resources:

ALL-NATURAL BIRD FOOD. *Wings* has created the first super-premium all natural, fortified food for wild birds, as well as a cage and aviary (pet) bird food line. *Wings* wild bird food was created in cooperation with (and has become the official bird food of) the NWF, National Wildlife Federation. *Wings* pet bird food was developed by well-known aviculturist/zoologist, Dr. Matthew M. Vriends and nutritionist B.F. (Brad) Batte. *Wings* is the highest quality bird food available, using only the best seeds while incorporating amino acids, antioxidants, enzymes, vitamins and minerals, Spirulina and Lactobacillus acidophilus. *Wings* contains no artificial ingredients and no fillers like rice, milo (sorghum), "grain products" and other undesirable fillers found in many bird food mixes. *Wings* is sold in health food stores, pet stores, eco stores, select grocery stores, specialty outlets, and major drug store chains across North America. WINGS/NATURAL WORLD INTERACTIONS, INC. P.O. Box 676, Oyster Bay, NY 11771-0676, (800)-WINGS-67, or 516-922-5987; FAX 516-922-4199

CRYSTALLOID MINERALS (electrolytes) FOR BODY AND SKIN. Trace minerals in crystalloid form allow for greater cellular absorption. **PetLyte™** puts the life force back in food and water to fortify the body's defense against chemical additives. It is a liquid blend of trace minerals in an electrolyte base **Skin-Aide™** is the first pet skin healing and nutrient spray,. Due to its crystalloid nature, its penetrates rapidly to the deepest skin layers with minerals and a unique blend of ionically bound herbs. NATURE'S PATH., P.O. Box 7862, North Port, FL 34287 (800)-326-5772

DR. HALLIDAY'S HIGH ENDURANCE AND HEALTH PRODUCTS. A superb energy supplement that includes electrolyte trace minerals, silica, biotin, etc. Easy to assimilate for birds and other pets. For complete product catalog contact NUTRANIMAL, 7974 Parkside Ct., Jenison, MI 49428 (888)-NUTRITION (Portion of proceeds go to Save the Black Rhino Foundation).

A LITTLE BIT OF EVERYTHING. Chemical free living is what every pet hopes their owner will give them. The **Whiskers mail order catalog** and store offers a multitude of natural and holistic products from food to frisbees, halters to homeopathy and everything in between. They are dedicated to providing you with safe, non-toxic alternatives to the products you may currently be using. For a free catalog call WHISKERS, 235 E 9th St., New York, NY 10003 (800)-944-7537 or (212)-979-2532 Web: *http://choicemall.com/whiskers*

CUSTOM ELECTROLYTE FORMULA. This **Custom Electrolyte Formula** with balanced ratios of all minerals essential for optimum health, helps to prevent dehydration and maintains proper fluid balance in the blood and tissues, stabilizes energy levels, combats fatigue, nausea, diarrhea and upset stomach and is good for nervous birds. NUTRI-PET RESEARCH, INC. 8 W. Main St., Farmingdale, NJ 07727 (800)-360-3300, (908)-938-2233.

ALL-NATURAL HIGH POTENCY DIGESTIVE ENZYMES. PROZYME™ is a highly concentrated blend of the most potent *plant source enzymes* available for improving digestion. **PROZYME** is scientifically proven to increase the bio-availability and absorption of vitamins, minerals, essential fatty acids and other vital nutrients, especially Zinc, Selenium, Vitamin B6 and Linoleic. Backed by 20 yrs. of field research, **PROZYME** is beneficial and safe for dogs, cats,birds, ferrets, rabbits, horses. and exotics. PROZYME PRODUCTS, 6600 N. Lincoln Ave., Lincolnwood, IL 60645 (800)-522-5537

"NUTRI-TECH" THE ULTIMATE WATER FILTRATION SYSTEM. Carico International has developed a "POINT OF USE" system with a unique design that has no moving parts nor requires electricity. It incorporates a multi-stage technology including sub-micron ceramic and selective adsorbents to address all priority pollutants including micro-organisms. Comes with installation kit and video. CARICO INTERNATIONAL, 50 Lisbon Pl., Staten Island, NY 10306-2456 (888)-4CI-PURE (424-7873 or (718)-667-7022.

OMEGA 3 WITHOUT FISH OIL. FORTIFIED FLAX provides necessary essential fatty acids with the oil in flax seed. It is nature's richest source of Omega-3 and this ground whole flax seed also contains all essential amino acids, high fiber, complex carbohydrates, vitamins and minerals. This necessary supplement comes in meal form, and therefore is easy to sprinkle on or mix into your pet's food. OMEGA-LIFE, Inc., P.O. Box 208, Brookfield WI 53008-0208 (800)-EAT-FLAX (328-3529).

SPIRULINA FOR PETS. Scientists in the USA, Japan, China, Russia and other countries are studying this safe blue-green algae to unlock its full potential. Current research indicates that **Spirulina** regresses tumors, prevents cancers, treats viral diseases and regulates immune system function by strengthening the body's own DNA repair processes. Feathers become soft and shiny. Skin irritations clear up. Infections may be prevented or respond better to treatments. Anemia, poisoning and immunodeficiency can be alleviated. Excellent for birds. EARTHRISE ANIMAL HEALTH, P.O. Box 459, Tollhouse, CA 93667 (800)-995-0681

SEAWEEDS & MICRONUTRIENTS FOR BIRDS. SOURCE® (nutritional micronutrients derived from seaweeds), has greatly benefited birds, with users reporting more intense coloration, stronger resilient feathers, improved shell strength and live hatch survival rates. SOURCE, INC., 101 Fowler Rd., N. Branford, CT 06471 (800)-232-2365

FULL SPECTRUM LIGHTING. This type of lighting is the closest to natural sunlight. It provides pet with a natural bright light and heat source that closely mimics the spectrum of natural sunlight. The extra long life **Lumichrome** bulb emits beneficial Ultraviolet rays. This type of lighting is essential to preventing depression in kennels and homes during the winter. M. PENCAR ASSOCIATES, 137-75 Geranium Ave., Flushing, NY 11355 (800)-788-5781

HOMEOPATHIC AND FLOWER REMEDIES. FDA registered, cruelty-free, 100% natural homeopathic pet treatments for anxiety, arthritis, cough, skin, trauma, urinary infections and incontinence, are available from **Homeopet.** The calming essence and non-addictive effectiveness of flower remedies is well documented. These creams and liquids relieve emotional stress and imbalances, and can act as excellent first aid products. BAYSIDE QUALITY PRODUCTS, 315 Franklin Ave., 2nd FL., Franklin Square, NY 11010 (888)-724-5489

NATURAL PET RELAXANT. Veterinarians recommend **Pet Calm** to relax and calm pets during stressful times such as boarding, traveling, storms and fireworks. Valerian is the main ingredient in **Pet Calm.** It has been used as a natural remedy for nervousness since ancient Greece. **Vita•Treat** pet care professionals produce 100% natural products for dogs, cats, birds and reptiles. VITA•TREAT, (800)-929-0418 (WA.)

HOMEOPATHIC DIGESTIVE AIDS & DETOXIFIERS. Healing animals is simple, safe and effective with homeopathic medicine. The **NEWTON P25 Digestive Aid** is a detoxifier formula for the liver of small animals such as cats, dogs, ferrets and birds. These formulas promote general body cleansing to speed the healing process and maintain good health and can be combined with other formulas to safely treat many common ailments that affect animals today. The Detoxifier is available for people too. NEWTON LABORATORIES, INC., 2360 Rockaway Ind. Blvd., Conyers, GA 30207 (800)-448-7256 E-mail: newtrmdy@avana.net

GARLIC EXTRACT. .More than 100 scientific studies have confirmed the safety and efficacy of the world's only truly odorless garlic. **KYOLIC® AGED GARLIC EXTRACT's.™** unique aging process brings out safer, more valuable and effective components than those in fresh raw garlic. Only **KYOLIC®** has anti-viral properties and anti-cancer activity, is truly a cell protector and helps activate the Phase II detoxifying enzymes system. WAKUNAGA OF AMERICA, CO., LTD., 23561 Madero, Mission Viejo, CA 92691 (800)-825-7888

OXYGEN ENHANCEMENT FOR PET HEALTH. EN GARDE Health Products is a pioneer in oxygen products, oxygen enhancement and products with sublingual application. Their human product **OXY-MOXY,** sublingual respiratory oxygen enhancer, was modified for cats (**OXY-CAT**), dogs, (**OXY-DOG**). The original **OXY-MOXY** can be used on birds, horses, & fish. EN GARDE HEALTH PRODUCTS, INC., PET DIVISION, 7702-10 Balboa, Van Nuys CA 91406 (800)-955-4633 (818)-901-8505 (to order) SSAE #10 for catalog.

BARLEY GRASS-SPIRULINA SUPPLEMENT. Malnutrition is the number one cause of death among caged exotic birds. prevent dietary deficiency with Barley Bird™, the "original" Spirulina-Barley Grass nutritional supplement. Sprinkle it on soft food and/or seeds as the convenient way to provide the much-needed raw vegetable nutrition in your bird's diet. Barley Bird features live plant enzymes for improved digestion of commercial foods, beta carotene, detoxifying chlorophyll, antioxidant vitamins, trace minerals, B vitamins, proteins and more. GREEN FOODS CORPORATION, Orders (800)-222-3374 (ext 434); Questions (800)-777-4430.

WATER FILTERS FOR YOUR PET'S HEALTH. Aqua Belle supplies a full line of residential water purifiers provide protection from lead, chlorine, certain bacteria, fluoride and sediment. Their extruded 4 stage carbon filters out perform carbon block and granular activated carbon filters (GAC) and come as whole house filters, countertop or under the sink point-of-use filters. This is a practical, inexpensive way to protect your pet from ill health due to water contamination. AQUA BELLE MFG. CO., P.O Box 496, Highland Park, IL 60035 (800)-243-2790, (847)-432-8979

RECYCLED NEWSPAPER LITTER. Canbrands International Ltd., has been manufacturing **Yesterday's News® Cat Litter and Small Animal & Bird Bedding** from recycled newspaper since 1987. All our products are non-toxic and contain an all natural odor controlling ingredient that neutralizes ammonia on contact. **Yesterday's News®** is dust free, will not track around the house or stick to the tray and will not stain. CANBRANDS INTERNATIONAL LTD. Sales & Marketing (800)-267-5287 E-mail: canbrand@nbnet.nb.

Bibliography.

-Cummings, Stephen, M.D. Ullman, Dana, M.P.H. *Everybody's Guide To Homeopathic Medicines*, Tarcher/Putnam Pub., New York, NY: 1991.

-Dean, Dr. Carolyn *Complementary Natural Prescriptions for Common Ailments*, Keats Pub., New Canaan, CT: 1994.

-Chapman, Beryl M. *Homeopathic Treatment For Birds*, C.W Daniel Company Limited, Great Britain, 1991.

-Day, Christopher *The Homeopathic Treatment of Small Animals; Principles And Practice*, C.W. Daniel Company Limited, Great Britain, 1992.

-Boericke, William, M.D. *Materia Medica with Repertory*, Boericke & Tafel, Inc., Santa Rosa, CA, 1927.

-Balch, James, M.D. Balch, Phyllis A., C.N.C. *Prescription for Nutritional Healing*, Avery Pub. Group Inc., Garden City Park, NY, 1990.

-Somer, Elizabeth M.A., R.D. *The Essential Guide to Vitamins and Minerals*, HarperCollins Pub., NY, NY,1992.

-oyle, Patrick G Jr. *Understanding the Life of Birds*, Summitt Pub., Lakeside, CA,1987.

-Kirschmann, Gayla J. and Kirschmann, John D., *Nutrition Almanac*, McGraw Hill, NY, NY, 1996.

-Santillo, Humbart, MH, N.D. *Food Enzymes* Holm Press, Prescott, AZ, 1993.

-Murray, Michael T., N.D. *The Healing Power of Foods*, Prima Pub. Rocklin, CA, 1993.

-Winter, Ruth, M.S. *Medicines In Food*. Crown Trade Paperbacks, New York, 1995.

-Lewis, Walter H. & Memory, Elvin-Lewis P.F., *Medical Botany*, Wiley-Interscience Pub., New York, 1977.

-Marderosian, Ara Der, Ph.D., Liberti, Lawrence E., M.S., *Natural Product Medicine*, Stickley, Philadelphia, PA, 1988.

-Burton Goldburg Group *Alternative Medicine*, Washington: Future Medicine Pub., Puyallup, 1993.

-Lau, Benjamin, M.D., Ph.D. *Garlic Research Update*, Canada: Odyssey Publishing Inc., Vancouver, B.C., 1991.

-Chaitow, Leon and Trenev, Natasha, *Probiotics*, Thorsons Publishers, Hammersmith, London, 1990.

-Crook, William G., M.D., *The Yeast Connection*, Vintage Books, New York: 1986.

Mitsuoka, Tomotari, Ph.D. *Intestinal Bacteria and Health*, Tokyo, Japan: H.B.J. Japan,1978.

-Schmidt, Michael A., Smith, Lendon H., Sehnert, Keith W. *Beyond Antibiotics*, North Atlantic Books, Berkeley, CA, 1993.

-Steiner, Charles V., Jr., D.V.M and Davis, Richard B., D.V.M., M.S. *Caged Bird Medicine*, Iowa State University Press, Ames, Iowa, 1981.

-Linder, Maria C., Ph.D. *Nutritional Biochemistry and Metabolism*. Appleton and Lange, Norwalk, CT:, 1991.

-Tyler, Varro E., Ph.D., Sc.D. *Herbs of Choice*, Pharmaceutical Products Press, Bingamton, NY, 1994.

-Graham, Judy *Evening Primrose Oil*, Healing Arts Press, Rochester, VT, 1989.

INDEX

disaccharides, 24
dolomite, 33
dry skin, 4, 29, 30, 31, 37

—E——F—

E. coli, 59
echinacea, 18, 40, 50
elastin, 35
electrolyte, 34, 45, 52, 66
enzymes, 1, 3, 9, 16, 17, 18, 20, 24, 25, 26, 29, 33, 34, 35, 40, 58, 60, 61, 66, 67, 68, 69
essential amino acids, 12, 25, 26, 67
essential fatty acids, 1, 12, 21, 52, 67
Euphrasia, 43
evening primrose oil, 27, 52
fats, 25, 26, 28, 29, 33, 46, 47, 60
feather loss, 4, 27, 28, 34
feathers, 25, 27, 28, 29, 30, 31, 34, 35, 37, 45, 46, 67
flax seed oil, 52, 55
flower essence, 51
fracture, 44
free radicals, 28, 29, 36
fried foods, 23
fructose, 55

—G—

garlic, 16, 18, 29, 30, 33, 34, 36, 54, 59, 62, 68
Giardia, 63
gizzard, 60
glucosinolates, 21
glycoalkaloid, 22
goiter, 14, 21, 35
goitrogenic glycosides, 21
goldenseal, 50, 63
gout, 22, 26, 27, 29, 30, 31, 54, 55, 59
Gram's stain, 61
grapefruit extract, 40, 50

—H——I—

handfeeding, 51, 56, 58, 60, 61, 62

heart, 27, 29, 30, 31, 32, 33, 34, 36, 54
hemicellulose, 25
herbal, 41, 43, 45, 50, 51, 62, 63
homeopathy, 42, 66
hydrochloric acid, 33, 34
hyperactivity, 48
hypercalcemia, 32
Hypericum, 44
hypervitaminosis, 9, 28, 31
hypocalcemia, 33
hypothyroidism, 28, 35, 39, 54
hypovitaminosis, 10
Ignatia, 44
immune system, 8, 9, 14, 16, 21, 27, 28, 29, 31, 35, 36, 38, 39, 46, 47, 49, 50, 55, 57, 58, 59, 61, 63, 64, 67
infertility, 31
infusion, 43, 50, 51, 62
iodine, 14, 17, 21
iron, 14, 28, 29, 33, 35, 36

—K——L—

kava kava, 50
keratin, 25, 34
kidney disorders, 30
Klebsiella, 59
lectins, 20
lemon balm, 50
lima beans, 20
linoleic acid, 27
linolenic acid, 27
liver, 4, 24, 25, 26, 28, 29, 31, 34, 35, 36, 39, 54, 55, 59, 60, 63, 64, 68

—M——N—

magnesium, 16, 17, 18, 32, 33, 34, 52
malabsorption, 31
maldigestion, 24, 29
Manganum Aceticum, 44
mash, 12, 13, 16, 17, 18, 51
monosaccharides, 24
natural antibiotics, 61
Neomycin, 59